"Yael Calhoun's masterful understanding and passion for working with those who have experienced trauma are put forward in an easy and digestible way for anyone interested in working with this population. This is a must-read for anyone in the field of trauma-informed care."

**Brandon Yabko, PhD**, *licensed psychologist, SLC Psych, LLC*

"This science-based and comprehensive book is offered with compassion and deep knowledge from the life work of Yael Calhoun, a leader in the field of trauma-informed yoga."

**Denise Druce, C-IAYT**, *school director, Yoga Assets*

"Yael Calhoun's new book is a much-needed resource that weaves together the latest science, traditional practices, and the knowledge of an experienced teacher and yoga expert who understands trauma. Her practical tips such as 'show, don't tell' provide invaluable guidance and the skill-based chapters, including 'Suggested Breath Work' provide simple tools that can be used in a wide range of settings."

**Linda Chamberlain, PhD, MPH**

"Yael Calhoun's book is a useful resource for clinicians who wish to add yoga to their healing and stress reduction toolkit. The book helps bring the ancient practice of yoga to help us today with our increasing awareness of the toxicity of life traumas and the need for many ways to address them. Thank you, Yael!"

**David L. Corwin, MD**, *professor of pediatrics and director of forensic services at the University of Utah*

"This book is a gift. It is a beautiful scientific and empathetic guide to helping healers heal some of the most vulnerable human beings in our communities."

**Mara L. Rabin, MD**, *medical director, Utah Health and Human Rights*

"Yael Calhoun has concisely and uniquely blended the essential concepts of neuroscience with mindfulness and yoga-based practices to both educate and empower the individual toward robust healing. She is brilliant in descriptions and effective in guidance toward resolution and resilience. What a gift her work is to any and all in recovery—and we are all in recovery from one thing or another!"

**Susie Wiet, MD**, *founder and medical director of Sovegna, founder of Trauma Resiliency Collaborative, and board member of the Academy on Violence and Abuse*

"*Building Safety with Trauma-Informed Yoga* is full of valuable gems not only for those teaching yoga but for all therapists working with traumatized populations. Yael Calhoun offers practical tools delivered with compassion and wisdom. Her book is a gift to the field and the result of her years of exquisite work!"

**Lori S. Katz, PhD**, *author of* Holographic Reprocessing for Healing Trauma, Abuse and Maltreatment

"*Building Safety with Trauma-Informed Yoga* is an insightful, inspiring and practical guide for anyone who works with people who have experienced trauma. Grounded in the science of traumatic stress, the reader is given the context, the language, and direction necessary to provide a safe yoga space and experience for even the most traumatized of individuals. The book does not proselytize yoga or trauma-informed care, rather it grounds the reader in the science of how trauma impacts both the mind and the body and then clearly articulates how trauma-informed yoga can impact the mind through movement and breath to enhance resilience. After reading this book you won't just know the right things to say to make someone feel safe, but much more importantly, you will have a better sense of what to do to allow them to feel safe. This is really a must-read book for yoga professionals who want to be trauma-informed as well as non-yoga trauma professionals who want to expand and develop their interdisciplinary capacity to work collaboratively with yoga professionals."

**Brooks Keeshin, MD**, *child abuse pediatrician and child psychiatrist*

"What makes this trauma-informed yoga guidebook so remarkable is that it is grounded in science and written by a teacher who draws on decades of experience teaching yoga to people who have experienced trauma. Calhoun's insights, scope, and practice can be incorporated into trauma-informed healthcare and educational institutions as part of an evidence-based additional healing modality."

**Tasneem Ismailji MD, MPH**, *co-founder and board member of the Academy on Violence and Abuse*

"Yael Calhoun offers a scrupulous and comprehensive overview of trauma and the application of yoga practices for addressing its associated symptoms in this book. It is superbly written and richly referenced with quotes from many trauma therapists, clinicians, and researchers. I consider it a very valuable resource for teachers providing therapeutic yoga practices including those for trauma."

**James Fox**, *founding director of the Prison Yoga Project*

"As yoga teachers, we do not know all our students' personal stories. But it's highly likely that one or more of our students have experienced some sort of trauma. Our words, tone of voice and practice methods all matter. Yael Calhoun's compassion and extensive experience in working with trauma shine through in this book. With its thorough and easily digested theory and practice suggestions, this book will help all yoga teachers create a safe, empowering environment for their students."

**Charlotte Bell**, *author of* Mindful Yoga, Mindful Life: A Guide for Everyday Practice *and* Hip-Healthy Asana: The Yoga Practitioner's Guide to Protecting the Hips and Avoiding SI Joint Pain

"An excellent resource for any yoga teacher keen to learn effective ways to guide trauma-informed recovery and resiliency-building skills."

**Rob Schware, PhD**, *executive director of Give Back Yoga Foundation*

# Building Safety with Trauma-Informed Yoga

*Building Safety with Trauma-Informed Yoga* is an accessible, science-based guide for clinicians, yoga teachers, teachers in training, and practitioners. The book provides clear ideas on how to support diverse groups in trauma recovery and in building resiliency skills. The easy-to-follow format is organized around the three key principles of building safety, supporting empowerment, and maintaining simplicity. Readers will find free downloadable support materials on the author's website, including handouts, flyers, scripts, and audio and video recordings.

**Yael Calhoun, MS, MA, E-RTY**, is the author or series editor of more than 20 books and manuals, including *Trauma-informed Yoga for Pain Management: A Practical Manual for Simple Stretching, Gentle Strengthening, and Mindful Breathing*. Yael is the executive director of GreenTREE Yoga®, a nonprofit dedicated to bringing the benefits of yoga to underserved populations and to those who work with them (www.greentreeyoga.org).

# Building Safety with Trauma-Informed Yoga

## A Practical Guide for Teachers and Clinicians

Yael Calhoun

Routledge
Taylor & Francis Group

NEW YORK AND LONDON

Designed cover image: Danny Breuker © Getty Images.

First published 2024
by Routledge
605 Third Avenue, New York, NY 10158

and by Routledge
4 Park Square, Milton Park, Abingdon, Oxon, OX14 4RN

*Routledge is an imprint of the Taylor & Francis Group, an informa business*

ISBN: 9781032308401 (hbk)
ISBN: 9781032308418 (pbk)
ISBN: 9781003308836 (ebk)

DOI: 10.4324/9781003308836

Typeset in Goudy
by Deanta Global Publishing Services, Chennai, India

To my family, far and wide, past and present, who taught me about trauma … and more importantly, about resiliency.

To Gina Jensen, LCSW, a beautiful example of resilience and a dedicated trauma warrior, taken from us much too soon.

To all those working to find peace in their lives and to those who support that work.

# Contents

# Acknowledgments

This book truly took a village of varied and wonderful individuals. Charlotte Bell, E-RYT, author and yoga teacher extraordinaire, was my first teacher 30 years ago. Had she not created such a welcoming practice, I probably would not have taken another yoga class. Her continued support of my projects has been invaluable. Nicole Cavallaro's enthusiasm and boundless energy provided a strong foundation as we cofounded GreenTREE Yoga® in 2007. Charlotte is a founding and current board member. The dedicated GreenTREE Yoga board has provided program support for over 15 productive years. Gina Jensen, LCSW, shepherded the trauma-informed yoga program at the Salt Lake City Veterans Administration, Utah, because she said I was so excited about trauma-informed yoga, she got excited. Many veterans came to my classes, and we learned together as I fine-tuned the program that grew to six classes a week. A special thanks to Cindy Silver, Siegrun Elisabeth Scorup, Joann Haines, Stacey Scott, and Angela M. Provstgaard, who attended our classes for years and who each, in unique ways, helped create a nurturing, supportive place for so many to connect, to be heard, and to laugh.

Many professionals have shared their talent and expertise. Yvette Melby, LCSW, RYT, and I collaborated and developed trauma-informed yoga programs for refugees, translated into six languages. A special thanks to all the wonderful participants in my workshops, classes, and trainings who have provided the invaluable questions and feedback that inspired this book. I am grateful to Margaret Clayton, PhD, APRN, FAAN, Professor Emerita, College of Nursing, University of Utah, and to Mona Bingham, PhD, RN, a retired Army Nurse Corps Officer who attended my pain management classes for years, for their review of the science sections. Others who shared their time, talents, and expertise include Elizabeth Q. Finlinson, LCSW (trauma therapist, our yoga model, and a founding GreenTREE Yoga® board member);

Cameron E. Hatch, LCSW (clinical social worker); and Katelyn D. O'Farrell, PhD, (exercise physiologist and yoga teacher). A special thanks to Denise Druce, E-RTY, for the amazing opportunity to teach the incarcerated (www .yogaassets.com). A group of dedicated yoga teachers, all working with trauma recovery, spent many hours reading the text, practicing the sequences, teaching the program, and sharing their insights. Your boots-on-the-ground contributions are more than you will ever know. Thank you, Rebecca Carroll, RYT 500; Mariann Bourland; Emma Powell, Amy Johnson, E-RYT, and Yvette Melby, LCSW, RYT. As I continue to say; "Teamwork." Finally, a very warm thanks to Sam Tresco for insisting he understood the concepts before doing his clear and inviting artwork (www.whitegorgedesigns.com).

# Preface

This book grew out of many years of developing and presenting workshops to teachers, clinicians, health care providers, and diverse groups working to recover from traumas. Then I expanded my program to provide trauma-informed certifications. Over the years, the materials for the workshops, which were offered for various professional education credits and presented nationally, grew as people requested more information. They wanted more science on trauma and yoga, written scripts, and class sequences. As I was sending out workshop information, it struck me that an easy-to-use book format, rather than pages of attachments, would have more value.

Like many, my interest in trauma was rooted in trying to understand the people in my life. My interest in neuroscience grew as both the trauma and yoga pieces came together. I did a training with David Emerson, author of *Overcoming Trauma Through Yoga*. I was so inspired by what I learned that I worked with a forward-thinking social worker, Gina Jensen, LCSW, at the Salt Lake VA to start a trauma-informed yoga veterans' program in 2011, which over ten years we built to six classes a week. Yvette Melby, LCSW, RYT, a multilingual social worker and yoga teacher who participated in the Bridging Borders Program, and I collaborated to develop a program for staff and refugees in Thai/Burmese camps. Those program materials have been translated into six languages and are used to train refugee women community leaders. Other groups I have taught include children who have experienced trauma; survivors of sexual assault; the incarcerated; and the staff at many hospitals, refugee centers, counseling/treatment centers, and domestic violence organizations.

In 2007, I co-founded GreenTREE Yoga, a nonprofit dedicated to bringing the healing benefits of yoga to underserved populations and to those professionals who work with them (www.greentreeyoga.org). A founding board member, Elizabeth Q. Finlinson, LCSW, a gifted trauma therapist, worked tirelessly with me to shape our trauma-informed programs, all of which have guided the writing of this book. In the spirit of full disclosure, my educational and professional background inform my approach. I have taught college science courses and was a municipal environmental planner focusing on water issues. I like a strong, system-based plan based on solid science.

My intention is to bring the ideas that shaped my trauma-informed programs together, using my own teaching experiences as a guide to illustrate key principles. By providing a strong base of what works, I want to support your efforts to create a program that meets your personal and professional needs. As an example, consider these three phrases I use in my trainings. People say they hear them later as they are sharing yoga, whether a two-minute break in a clinical or health care setting or a full practice. The first phrase is 'Trust the Yoga'. Instead of explaining everything, you are creating an opportunity for someone to experience in their own way the benefits of yoga. The phrase 'Show, Don't Tell' speaks to the need that many teachers and clinicians have to share all they have learned. Instead of explaining the reasons for and the benefits of getting grounded, show someone with specific grounding breathwork and movements. My third phrase is relevant to anyone sharing yoga: 'Stay in Your Lane'. Be a yoga purist by keeping the yoga time, whether a 1-minute break or a 90-minute class, about doing yoga.

These ideas support three goals in being trauma-informed: building safety, supporting empowerment, and maintaining simplicity. If you 'Trust the Yoga', if you 'Show, Don't Tell', and if you 'Stay in Your Lane', you can greatly simplify your methods, as you guide someone to the place in which they are able to, as Victor Frankl said, "choose one's attitude in any given set of circumstances, to choose one's own way."

# Introduction

## Introduction

This book is a practical guide to using the body-based modality of yoga for trauma recovery and for building resiliency skills. While it is written for those who want to share trauma-informed yoga, it also may be helpful to individuals looking for more information on trauma recovery tools. The ideas in this book can help explain someone's responses, minimize guilt and shame, and support trauma recovery efforts. It can be a strong starting point from which to grow your current program and meet your personal and professional needs. This book presents ideas on how to develop a trauma-informed skill set to manage what you can, to adjust for what you cannot control, and to have the awareness to know the difference. And, true to the heart of yoga, the book stresses the role of the breath as a healing and strengthening tool, which yogis have known based on thousands of years of empirical data. In short, this book explores the GreenTREE Yoga® Approach for building safety, supporting empowerment, and maintaining simplicity.

Let's consider what various experts have offered to define trauma and resiliency. Bessel van der Kolk, MD, says trauma is losing one's way in the world. He reminds us that in 1889 Pierre Janet, MD, said: "Traumatic stress is an illness of not being able to be fully alive in the present" (van der Kolk, 2015). I think of a boat becoming unmoored as you lose connections to yourself, your family, your community, and the world. Not being present means one may be stuck somewhere else, perhaps stuck in fragments of the past, unable to move forward. Dr. Janet also wrote about these traumatic fragments or residues intruding on behavior in the present (van der Kolk, 1989). As Gabor Maté, MD, says in his book, *The Myth of Normal*, "Trauma isn't something that happens to you, it happens *inside* of you" (Mate, 2022). Trauma can be from

DOI: 10.4324/9781003308836-1

a single event or from the cumulative effects of multiple traumatic events, called complex trauma, as discussed in the ACES studies (Felitti, 1998). Dr. Maté notes, what traumas have in common is they involve a "fracturing of self and one's relationship to the world" (Maté, 2022).

Today we have a better understanding of what can cause these traumatic memory fragments and how to integrate them to create a coherent, nondisruptive narrative. It makes sense that trauma recovery protocols are based on helping someone reconnect – first with themselves, then with others, and with their environment. Peter Levine, PhD, says "Trauma can be prevented or transformed" (Levine, 2010). Preventing trauma speaks to someone's ability to bounce back and to reestablish connections after trauma stress. We call this skill resiliency, which comes from the Latin *resiliēns* meaning to leap or to spring back. Dr. Levine talks about somatically based steps to move someone from paralysis to transformation. This book offers body-based tools to support efforts to reconnect and to build resiliency skills.

Now we can consider what trauma-informed means. Trauma-informed yoga is not a specific type of yoga as are Ashtanga, Kundalini, Hatha, vinyasa, or restorative. Rather, trauma-informed is an approach that can be applied to many styles. Trauma-informed means someone is informed about the possible effects of trauma, so as not to trigger or stress people in recovery. As many key therapists state, it is not necessary to know the type of trauma someone has suffered, as they may not even be able to put it into words. Trauma-informed practitioners, including teachers, clinicians, and health care professionals, can hone their skills in reading body language, which is really telling some of the story. As Pat Ogden, PhD, says, "… use the body as an entry point to the emotions" (Ogden, 2006). This point is not trivial. Teachers, clinicians, and health care providers may never learn the details of a trauma, yet they can still provide trauma-informed, essential help. Consider that trauma-informed certifications offered to such organizations as schools and shelters are to educate staff about shaping policies and responding to situations in a trauma-informed way. It is not about individualized therapy.

Several themes are interwoven throughout the book. One is science, which rightly claims the first chapter. The intention is both to inspire and to inform your teaching, clinical work, or personal efforts to heal through discussions on the science of trauma and yoga. In addition, three key principles comprise the other themes: building safety, supporting empowerment, and maintaining simplicity. These themes provide the structure for chapters on breathwork and the yoga practice. As I thought about the best way to share what I have learned through my studies and my teaching, the way to organize this book became clear.

**Chapter 1:** The first chapter must be the science. You already may have an interest in how your brain works, the mind/body connection, and why it matters, so this chapter is for you. Or perhaps you return to this chapter later. A 45-minute narrated PowerPoint is available in three formats: a transcript, an MP3, and an MP4 (Appendix C: Supplemental Resources). Please note the ideas are based on the research and writings of many key trauma researchers and practitioners. The questions that frame this chapter are: Are we stuck? Why is a sense of safety important? Where does a sense of safety come from? What does trauma do to that sense of safety? The last section discusses the science of breathwork and of movement, putting it all together in the final question: why can trauma-informed yoga help someone to get unstuck? 'Be informed and be inspired'.

**Part I: Preparing to Teach:** It was logical that the next section should be about how someone prepares to teach, whether a yoga break or a full practice. Being trauma-informed does not mean everything has to be just right in your space. Rather, it means you begin with a strong plan and learn to work with what you have in a predictable and consistent way. The chapters on language, the yoga space, and classroom management introduce practical tools organized around three themes: again, building safety, supporting empowerment, and maintaining simplicity. I have had many teachers and clinicians say to me, "Oh, that makes sense. I hadn't thought of that." The ideas may be a guide but also may provide a seed crystal, prompting you to think of your own examples or applications.

As I put together my notes for the book, it was clear that there were many considerations specifically for teachers, clinicians, and health care professionals. Turns out the ideas filled Chapter 5. Personal qualities, personal challenges (including self-care), ways to incorporate yoga into any setting, and ways to practice how you teach are discussed.

**Part II: Teaching Protocols:** The ideas in Part 1 (language, the space, and what's done in the space) set the foundation for Part II. Breathwork is not an extra in a yoga class. It is an integral part of the practice, so it is fitting that the breath commands two chapters. Chapter 6 considers *why* breathwork should be a key part of your program. Chapter 7 is framed around the idea that because breathwork is a key part of any yoga practice, *how* you teach breathwork is a key part of any yoga practice. It organizes breathwork into easy-to-use sections, complete with scripts, variations, and explanations about how the breathwork was developed. The format of considerations followed by applications continues in Chapters 8 and 9. Chapter 8 considers *why* a focus on simple breathwork and movement, your pacing, your use of language, and other factors can empower someone to widen their window of tolerance. The ideas in this chapter set a firm foundation for Chapter 9: *how* to plan and to teach your trauma-informed practice.

A very special chapter to me is Chapter 10, working with refugees and immigrants. The chapter includes considerations of language (English as a Second or Other Language, ESOL) cultural awareness, and social needs. Chapter 11 offers ideas on trauma-informed phrasing and practice sequences. Downloadable materials in various formats can support your efforts to grow a trauma-informed program (Appendix C: Supplemental Resources).

This book provides a detailed guide so your program can support building these skills:

- Using awareness of the breath and the body as a way to stay present.
- Learning to self-regulate using breath and movement.
- Activating the social engagement system.
- Learning to *feel* the body.
- Learning to tolerate bodily sensations by breathing and moving through sensations that could trigger.
- Becoming more open to processing using language.

It is my hope that the easy-to-follow format ensures this book's continued use as both a guide and reference as your programs evolve. This book provides a place to start and a place to practice and to learn. It is a place with a solid base of strong science and practical methods that work.

## References

Felitti, V. J., et al. (1998). The Adverse Childhood Experiences (ACE) Study. *American Journal of Preventive Medicine*, 14, 245–258.

Levine, Peter. (2010). *In an Unspoken Voice: How the Body Releases Trauma and Restores Goodness*. Berkeley: North Atlantic Books.

Maté, Gabor. (2022). *The Myth of Normal*. New York: Avery, pp. 20; 22.

Ogden, Pat. (2006). *Trauma and the Body: A Sensorimotor Approach to Psychotherapy*. New York: W. W. Norton and Company, p. 146.

Van der Kolk, Bessel A. (2015). *The Body Keeps the Score: Brain, Mind, and Body in the Healing of Trauma*. New York: Penguin Publishing, p. 312.

Van der Kolk, Bessel A., et al. (1989). Janet Pierre Janet and the Breakdown of Adaptation in Psychological Trauma. *American Journal of Psychiatry*, 146(12), 1530–1540.

# 1
# Science
## Be Informed and Be Inspired

At my workshops, clinicians, health care providers, and yoga teachers respond to the science component in one of two ways. Some want to understand the science and make their programs more intentional. They wanted more science. Others feel buoyed knowing the training is based on peer-reviewed research and might want more information later. Seeds have been planted. Therefore, this chapter is for everyone. A Brain Bonus based on this chapter is offered in three formats: a narrated PowerPoint (MP4) with eight ten-minute modules each including a yoga break, an audio file (MP3), and a transcript (Appendix C: Supplemental Resources). The GreenTREE Yoga® Approach for building safety, supporting empowerment, and maintaining simplicity is based on the many books and research cited throughout this book. While some are new, others are foundational works that will guide us for years.

Let's start with a question asked by the Harvard researcher, John Ratey, MD "Why should you care about how your brain works?" he asks in *Spark: The Revolutionary New Science of Exercise and the Brain.* His answer:

> Your life changes when you have a working knowledge of your brain. It takes guilt out of the equation when you recognize that there's a biological basis for certain emotional issues. On the other hand, you won't be left feeling helpless when you see how you can influence that biology.
>
> (Ratey, 2007/13)

With Dr. Ratey's ideas as our guide, let's consider the science behind these basic questions: Are we stuck? Why is a sense of safety important? Where does a sense of safety come from? What does trauma do to that sense of safety? These ideas lead to the final question: how can we use yoga to put it all together and empower someone to get unstuck?

DOI: 10.4324/9781003308836-2

## Are We Stuck?

Are people stuck in trauma without the possibility of moving ahead to build and to enjoy better lives? To answer this question and to be inspired by the possibilities, it is helpful to understand the science behind both trauma and the healing benefits of yoga. That is, as Dr. Ratey suggests, to "have a working knowledge of your brain."

## Neuroplasticity: Another Type of Plastic

Current brain imaging research supports what Sigmond Freud, Moshe Feldenkrais, William James, Ramón y Cajal, and others had studied since the late 1800s. In the 1890s, Dr. Cajal developed what he called the neural doctrine, something that has guided the science ever since. William James, MD, often called the father of psychology, coined the term plasticity, referring to the brain's ability to change. Today we call this property neuroplasticity. The research continues, underscoring the words of Sir Isaac Newton: "If I have seen a little further, it is by standing on the shoulders of Giants."

It is no longer thought that we are born hardwired, unable to change. Instead, neuroscience confirms that we are capable of real growth throughout our lifetimes because our brains can and do change. An engaging book that details these possibilities is *Livewired: The Inside Story of the Ever-changing Brain* by David Eagleman, PhD, a Stanford neuroscientist (Eagleman, 2020). More discussions on the science and heartening real life examples can be found in, *The Brain That Changes Itself: Stories of Personal Triumph from the Frontiers of Brain Science* by Norman Doidge, MD (Doidge, 2007). The 1990 Nobel Prize winner, Eric Kandel, MD, discusses how the biology of the mind, or that which bridges the sciences and the humanities, will improve our understanding of ourselves (Kandel, 2007). He discusses the research and tremendous implications of neural networks not being fixed in *In Search of Memory: The Emergence of a New Science of the Mind*.

From this renewed appreciation comes a profound sense of the possibilities in our abilities to empower someone to move toward better health. Western science continues to find evidence of what other cultures have understood for thousands of years, that connecting the mind and the body using the breath are key components in trauma recovery and in building resiliency. We are, quite simply, not stuck. Let's explore the basic body physiology that creates and supports these life-affirming connections.

## The Basics: All Systems Go

Let's start with a working definition of a neuron. Neurons are nerve cells found throughout the body: the brain, the skin, the muscles, and the organs, including the gut. In the brain alone, there are over 90 billion neurons (Zimmer, 2023). Fun neuron fact: 80 percent of the neurons found outside of the brain are in the gut. A review of the science will show why a gut feeling is actually real and how this fact relates to trauma. But first, back to the basics.

**What Makes a Neuron:** A neuron has several parts: the cell body, often called gray matter, contains the nucleus and DNA; the axons generate signals to other neurons; and, the dendrites receive signals (Figure 1.1). The axons, often called the white matter, are covered by myelin sheaths, fatty white material along the length of the neurons that can increase the speed at which neurons can fire by up to 3,000 times. As you practice something, myelin is one reason your proficiency increases. The spaces between the neurons are called the synapses. These basic facts will help clarify the later discussion of how neurochemical changes from stress and trauma can damage neurons.

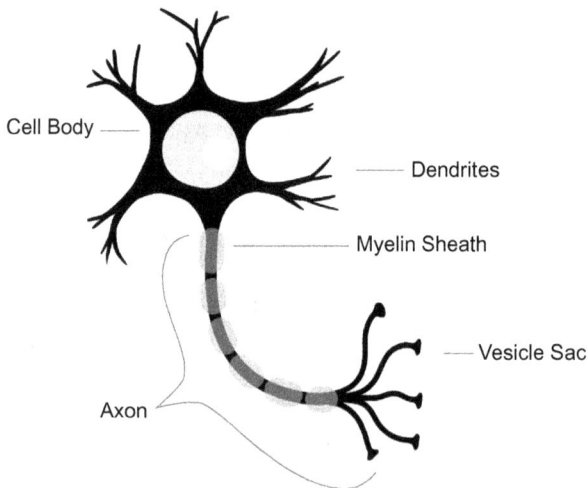

**Figure 1.1** A Neuron

**What Neurons Do:** Slamming on your brakes to avoid hitting a dog or running toward a child for a welcoming hug can happen because you first process information and then react. That processing and reacting happen as neurons send electrical and chemical signals throughout the body. Neurons are at-the-ready, having a store of chemical messengers, both neurotransmitters and hormones. These messengers are stored in the vesicle sacs and ready to be released into the synapses, the space between the neurons, and taken up by the dendrites of other neurons (Figure 1.2). Here is the point at which it gets really interesting. Messengers are not all the same, and messengers do not always do the same things. At various times, some speed things up, some slow things down, and some act to modulate responses. You may have heard of some of these chemical messengers: serotonin, cortisol, dopamine, and epinephrine (adrenaline). Books continue to be written on the topic, and research and discovery are ongoing.

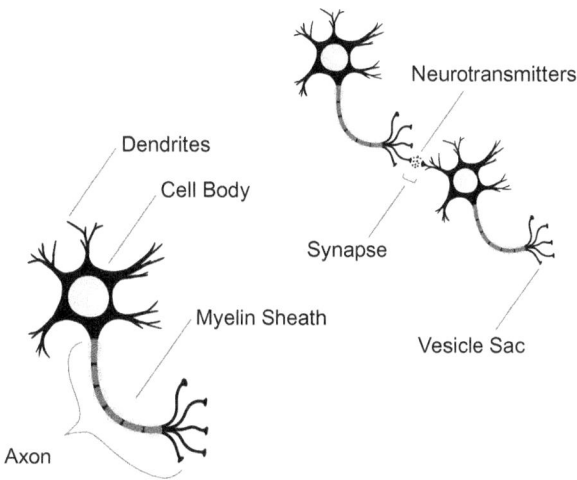

**Figure 1.2** Neuronal Connections

**All Neurons Are Not the Same:** Another fun neuron fact: among the 90 billion neurons in the brain, one of the smallest is about four microns. The longest neurons are in the sciatic nerve, with axons that can stretch over three feet from the base of the brain down each leg. Neurons can be sensory, relaying information from our senses in the form of electrical impulses. You are driving and see a toddler in the street, which is sensory information. You hit the brakes. These signals come from motor neurons, which control your muscle movements, both voluntary and involuntary. Did you have to think about hitting the brakes? Considering the answer provides more information relevant to trauma, which we will circle back to after a few more basics.

## The Nature/Nurture Debate: Who's Winning Now?

**Let's Talk About It:** Many lively philosophical discussions over the years have been fueled by the nature/nurture question: which is the stronger determining factor of who we are, our genetics or our environment? Today the question has evolved. We cannot change the hand we're dealt: our genetic make-up, for example, eye color and leg length, remains a constant. While CRISPR/Cas9 can edit specific genes, currently we are not designing human beings or deleting traumatic memories (Doudna, 2014). But science has shown we can change what we do with what we have. The Stanford neurobiologist Robert Sapolsky, PhD, offers a comprehensive look at why it misses the mark to rely solely on biology or on psychology/culture to explain human beings. His book, *Behave: The Biology of Humans at Our Best and Worst* (Sapolsky, 2018), is a must read for those who want to ponder more questions about the why of who we are. These new discussions focus on the dynamic interplay between our genetics and our experiences that continually shapes and reshapes our brains. This interplay is key in trauma recovery and in building resiliency skills.

**You've Got a Friend:** A large part of what happens to most of us involves our interactions with people. Daniel Siegel, MD, has devoted much of his research to the field of Interpersonal Neurobiology (IPNB), or how our connection with others and our ability to use others to self-regulate shape our brain. His many books provide insights and data into this emerging field (Siegel, 2012, 2020). You may feel bolstered knowing your efforts to connect with someone, whether as a teacher, a health care provider, or a friend, can help heal the brain. An interesting note: research continues to show the act of offering support to others also creates feelings of well-being in the helper (Dore, 2017).

## How Does Neuroplasticity Happen?

Let's go back to 1949 and an idea formalized by a Canadian researcher, Donald Hebb, MD. He stated that when we learn something, the connections between neurons become stronger and faster forming stronger neural networks. He termed the process use-dependent plasticity (Hebb, 1949). Carla Shatz, PhD, a groundbreaking Stanford neuroscientist, is credited with saying "neurons that fire together, wire together", with the corollary "neurons that fire out of sync, lose their link" (Shatz, 1992). Perhaps consider you are walking on a forest trail that is not well-travelled. It is slow walking with all the tree branches, roots, and rocks in the path. But then the trail becomes popular when a mile in someone finds a hot spring. Over time, more paths are worn, creating an even larger, more accessible trail system. Back to neurons making stronger connections by firing and then wiring together. Scientists observe that in a healthy brain, these neuronal connections grow stronger as they integrate and work together.

Back to the hot spring, which has grown cold and uninviting. With no one walking the trails, they become overgrown and impassable. Instead, you find a new trail to a waterfall, and well, you get the idea. As you think or act a new way, the old path, or the old neuronal connections, can weaken. Use it or lose it. You may be thinking, "Aha! I see how helpful to trauma recovery it could be for someone to be able to change how they respond to or think about something." Not only can someone learn new responses, but now clinicians are talking about unlearning other responses. Dr. Eric Kandel's research explored the idea of learned safety, looking at the neuroscience of how a sense of safety can be learned (Kandel, 2006). Pat Ogden, PhD, says, "We can't change what happened, but we can create new associations within that memory" (Ogden, 2007). Yoga philosophy has discussed these ideas for years. *Samskaras* are ways of unconsciously doing things again and again. The critical question in trauma recovery is how can change happen, and how can someone be a guide for that change? The answer comes as we keep exploring the neuroscience of trauma.

Dr. Eric Kandel's 1990 Nobel Prize–winning research showed two mechanisms create change: thought and experience. So not only what we think, but our experiences or what happens to us, can support neuroplastic changes in the brain throughout the lifespan. Dr. Kandel's interest in the science of memory is rooted in childhood experiences in Nazi-occupied Austria (Kandel, 2006). Research continues to show that large networks of interconnecting neurons are not fixed. Norman Doidge, MD, explores the science and offers many compelling examples in the book *The Brain's Way of Healing: Remarkable Discoveries and Recoveries from the Frontiers of Neuroplasticity* (Doidge, 2015). This book can inspire anyone interested in helping others or themselves to make meaningful life changes.

A couple of questions may come to mind. Are these brain changes always for the better? The short answer is these changes can be adaptive, as when someone learns a job skill. But changes can be maladaptive, as when someone becomes stuck in a highly reactive response to certain stimuli, whether actual or simply perceived. Yes, a trauma trigger is body physiology, a key idea found throughout this book. It is also an idea worth considering when thinking about feelings of guilt and shame that can be triggered by certain stimuli, perceived or real. Another question may be what physiological conditions support adaptive neuroplastic changes? Or quite simply, how do we get unstuck? Let's start at the beginning.

## Why Is a Sense of Safety So Important?

Why does Bessel van der Kolk, MD, say, "The single most important issue for traumatized people is to find a sense of safety in their own bodies" (van der

Kolk, 2015). Why does a feeling of safety support adaptive neuroplastic changes while being physiologically necessary to our mental and physical health?

## Getting Stuck

Science has shown that when you do not feel safe, your body secretes such stress hormones as cortisol, epinephrine (adrenaline), and norepinephrine. These elevated levels can get us out of bed in the morning, to work on time, and improve our job or school performance. Short-term spurts of cortisol and epinephrine can move us out of danger and toward safety. But long-term stress, or a chronic feeling of being unsafe or on high alert, means your body is continuously flooded with stress hormones. I saw a cartoon with a caption that said: "If you bark at everything, you can't go wrong." The clinical term for that set point is hypervigilance. This symptom is part of the post-traumatic stress disorder (PTSD) diagnosis, in which the body perceives continual danger and stays flooded with stress hormones. Joseph Ledoux, PhD, uses our instinctive response to a snake to illustrate someone stuck in a stress response. It may be a stick, but a hypervigilant person will continue to perceive and then respond to it as a snake (Ledoux, 2015). In addition to the laundry list of physical and mental health issues associated with chronic stress, a key problem relevant to trauma is chronic stress results in a greatly diminished ability to pay attention. 'It's body physiology'.

## Getting Unstuck: 'Pay Attention!'

The familiar cry of teachers and parents to 'Pay attention!' shows knowledge many of us have gained through experience. Neuroscience shows that if you cannot pay attention, you cannot learn new things, which includes learning new ways of processing stimuli. Okay, let's move from a well-worn hiking trail to a bookstore, one filled with self-help books promising 'Thirty Days to a Better You'. You buy the book, so it has your attention. You may do what it suggests for 30 days. What is happening here ? You are, in fact, rewiring your brain. Again, Dr. Kandel's Nobel Prize–winning science: thought and action can create changes. But there is more science to discuss.

There is a physiological reason why Dr. Daniel Siegel says, "Attention is the scalpel of neuroplasticity" (Siegel, 2012). He notes one key practical lesson of modern neuroscience is that how we direct our attention can shape how our brain works. Attention shapes how neurons fire, which in turn shapes the structure of the brain itself (Siegel, 2010). The physiological stage for rewiring the brain is set when we pay attention because certain neurotransmitters, like acetylcholine and norepinephrine, are released, setting up the release of more neurotransmitters involved in learning. Dopamine and glutamate also play roles. And again, we pay attention when something has salience or importance to us. You may be getting a sense of why this book starts with the basics of neurons. Spoiler alert: one of the most powerful things that a body-based yoga practice offers is an increased ability to pay attention, a result of body awareness and self-regulation skills. But learning new responses and unlearning other responses require that we feel safe enough to pay attention. This critical thread is woven through the remainder of this book. Let's consider what we mean by the physiology of safety.

## Where Does a Sense of Safety Come From?

This question of where a sense of safety comes from is not a casual one as our discussion will show. If we can grasp why a building sense of safety is the crux move, as the expression goes, we can be much more effective clinical and teaching guides. A.A. Milne, a veteran of WWI nerve gas trench warfare, wrote in *The House at Pooh Corner*: "'Pooh!' he whispered. 'Yes, Piglet?' 'Nothing,' said Piglet, taking Pooh's paw. 'I just wanted to be sure of you.'" Keep that in mind when we discuss the benefits of social support.

### To Coin a Phrase

Let's put the science in some historical context by looking at the phrase fight or flight. In the 1890s, Walter Cannon, MD, noticed that stress affected animals' digestive processes. In the 1920s he coined the term fight-or-flight and what he called the emergency reaction system. He also coined using the word homeostasis to mean a process by which biological systems maintain stability while adjusting to changing conditions (Cannon, 1929). This idea is the basis for understanding what self-regulation means.

Adding to this research is the now classic book by Hans Seyle, MD, *The Stress of Life* (Seyle, 1956). Dr. Seyle, an endocrinologist, coined the term stress to mean a response of the body to any demand, whether it is caused by, or results in, pleasant or unpleasant conditions. For years, it was thought that the nervous system was a simple on/off mechanism, an automatic function, not under conscious control. The autonomic nervous system has two branches. One branch is the sympathetic nervous system, mediating the fight, flight, or freeze response. Early research popularized stress as a negative to be kept in check by the other autonomic branch of the nervous system, the parasympathetic, sometimes called the rest-and-digest branch.

The foundational, peer-reviewed body of scientific work of Stephen Porges, PhD, on the polyvagal theory, is embraced and cited by many of the top trauma researchers and clinicians today. It expands our understanding of the nervous system and therefore lends clear guidance to anyone working in trauma recovery. His work has generated much research and many new protocols, putting the polyvagal theory front and center in clinical work today. To better appreciate how this theory builds on the older nervous system model, let's first step back to look at the bigger picture.

## The Triune Brain: The Bigger Picture

Let's look at basics of a healthy brain. The triune brain model was introduced in the 1960s by the neuroscientist and physician Paul Maclean, MD (Maclean, 1990) (Figure 1.3). Even at the time, he noted it was too simple a model owing to the great interconnectedness of brain structures. Yet the model provides a way to organize discussions about the three functional parts of the mammalian brain. (Sapolsky, 2017)

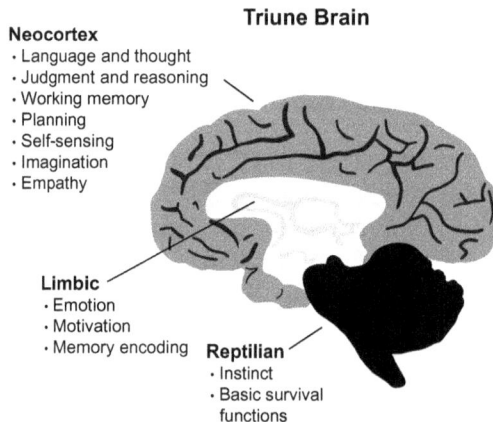

**Triune Brain**

**Neocortex**
· Language and thought
· Judgment and reasoning
· Working memory
· Planning
· Self-sensing
· Imagination
· Empathy

**Limbic**
· Emotion
· Motivation
· Memory encoding

**Reptilian**
· Instinct
· Basic survival functions

**Figure 1.3** The Triune Brain

**The Reptilian Brain – Simply Surviving:** The oldest part of the brain is the reptilian brain, sometimes called the lizard or the survival brain. The cerebellum (sometimes called the little brain) and the brain stem, regulate the body functions that keep us alive: eating, sleeping, digesting, reproducing, and both cardiac and respiratory functions. Current neuroscience continues to reveal more connections among the cerebellum and other parts of the brain. It's yet another example of the complex up–down connections or integration among many parts of the brain. Research and discovery are ongoing.

Our most primitive and instinctive response to danger is from the brainstem. That response is the immobilization or the freeze response. In humans, it can present as dissociation. Our bodies don't feel anything, so this instinctive response may save our lives. These responses do not require time to think and can numb feelings of intense pain. However, over time, responding without thought or feeling can prove maladaptive and even life-threatening.

I saw a photograph of a man's extended arm being slammed by a bat. Did he think, "Oh, this loose bat is really going to hurt," or "I cannot risk injury to my arm, I won't be able to work. So, do I want to do hurt my arm?" I would wager none of those thoughts went through his mind. In fact, I would wager that no thoughts went through his mind. His arm was extended in front of a young boy's head: instinctive survival response.

**The Limbic System – Getting All Emotional:** You most likely deal with the limbic system all day in the form of your emotions and those of others. The Latin root for emotion is *emovere*, which means to dislodge or to move out. The emotional brain gets us moving, either toward safety or pleasure or away from danger. Let's look at the four parts of a limbic model: the thalamus, the amygdala, the hypothalamus, and the hippocampus. We can then look at the ever-present stress feedback loops. This science may be new to you, or a refresher. Either way, taking some time with the basic science of emotions can guide how you empower someone, including yourself, to personalize their stress cycle. 'Be informed and be inspired'.

1. **Thalamus.** The thalamus is located above the brainstem and serves as a central relay station for many sensory and motor signals. How does the thalamus receive the signals in the first place? Does it matter? Yes. What we notice by hearing, taste, touch, and sight; how we tolerate what we notice; and, how this information gets conveyed to other parts of the brain are highly relevant to any trauma, resiliency, or pain discussion. The thalamus is the first stop. Pain is mentioned as pain and trauma can share neural pathways (Stanley, 2019; Maté, 2003). Did you notice that smell is not on the list? The only sensory signal not filtered through the thalamus is smell. We will revisit the significance of the neuroscience of smell in a trauma-informed setting, but examples relevant to your personal experiences already may have come to mind. The rest of this book discusses how to use these many sources of safety cues to your teaching advantage. Back to basics.

Signals sent to the thalamus come from within our body (wanting a snack or feeling your heart racing) and from outside our body (hearing the blaring horns or sounds of a stream). Signals are then sent to different brain areas: basic survival (reptilian), emotional (limbic), and neocortex (thinking). Stephen Porges offers a third type of cue, which he calls neuroception. Another recurring theme in this book is the need to be aware that someone's sense of safety is based on internal and external cues, from both conscious and unconscious sources. Let's look at the sources of information that shape our world.

- **Interoception – It's an Inside Job:** Interoception is our perception of bodily sensations (I feel tightness in my chest) and our awareness of our emotional states (I feel calm). Two areas in the neocortex that generate self-awareness signals are the insula and the medial prefrontal cortex, part of top-down processing discussed at the end of the chapter. William James talked about embodied cognition, the idea that emotions and related feelings arise from bodily cues (James, 1907). Given that 80 percent of the signals from the vagus nerve (discussed in the next section) travel from the body to the brain, the science fits. We know that 80 percent of the neurons outside of the brain line the gut and send signals, again, via the vagus nerve, to the brain (Porges, 2011). The gut has been dubbed the second brain. Current neuroscience continues to put to rest the 17th-century philosopher René Descartes' ideas on the mind and body being separate entities with the mind in control. "He felt gut-punched," or "It was heart-rending," are but two examples of vagal nerve science in common phrases. How is this science relevant to trauma recovery and building resiliency skills? Without self-awareness, the emotional brain lacks counsel from higher-level thinking. Studies continue to explore the findings that reduced interoception leads to low-stress thresholds or resiliency (Haase, 2016). The crucial role of interoception in recovery is another thread woven through this book.

- **Exteroception – It's an Outside Job!** We have another obvious source of information on which we rely to make our way in the world. Exteroception is the perception of sensations from stimuli outside the body. It could be from what we see, what we hear, what we taste, what we smell, or what we touch. The word perception comes from the Latin *perceptio*, meaning that which we collect or observe with our senses. Our perceptions are just that, ours. You see a mountain lion with a cub. Your perceptions may be shaped by being a photographer (career photograph) or a lost hiker (danger).

- **Neuroception – Below the Radar:** Our perceptions of stimuli can determine if we process something as safe or threatening. "Gotta grab my camera. This photo would make my article great," shows taking the time to think about actions and consequences. But, survival and emotional cues are processed more quickly because they do not use words. Dr. Stephen Porges coined the term neuroception to describe the process by which we detect these survival and emotional (subcortical) cues of safety (Porges, 2004). You may call it a sixth sense, intuition, or a gut feeling. You are consciously unaware of how you got that nonverbal information, yet you are able to process the signals and respond. Those signals (except for smell) have made their way to the thalamus. Joseph Ledoux, PhD, has called this form of processing the low road, as someone responds with speed not accuracy (Ledoux, 2015). You can probably guess what he terms the high road. The longer, more thoughtful processing route is from the thalamus to neocortex and then to the amygdala.

2. **Amygdala:** This structure is part of both scientific and philosophical discussions and books on aggression, fear, and anxiety (Sapolsky, 2017). Science shows that when we sense danger (real or perceived), sensory signals are sent from the thalamus to the amygdala to begin the fight, flight, or freeze response. Interestingly, the amygdala can receive some sensory information from the visual, auditory, and tactile cortex even before those signals have time to get processed in the cortex, higher level thinking. For example, you might see the grizzly bear (visual cortex), and your body responds before you even have time to think about it. Are you thinking or getting the feeling (or both) that brain science is complicated? Most would agree, so let's press on. Bessel van der Kolk calls the amygdala the smoke detector of the brain (van der Kolk, 2015). Once smoke is detected, the games begin. Responses, both conscious and subconscious, can happen quickly.

3. **Hypothalamus:** The hypothalamus secretes such necessary neurotransmitters as epinephrine (adrenaline), norepinephrine, and cortisol. To respond to threats, our muscles need increased levels of oxygen and glucose. Metabolic priorities shift from eating, resting, and reproducing, to the imminent, energy-intensive challenges of staying alive. Again, do we need to think this through? No, our perceptions signaling our rapid survival and emotional brain have us covered. Whether our perceptions are appropriate and adaptive or maladaptive is another question entirely, one highly relevant to any trauma discussion.

- **The HPA Axis – And Round and Round We Go:** Now let's look at the workings of someone's personal stress cycle, the hypothalamic–pituitary–adrenal (HPA) axis. Keep in mind that short-term stress stimulates the immune system, builds stress resiliency at the cellular level, and allows us to focus and to learn. Some have called short-term stress a form of stress inoculation. A note on the works of Dr. Seyle and Dr. Cannon in the 1900s: what both researchers clearly showed was abusing animals had clear, negative health effects, often resulting in death. More recent stress studies now consider the adaptive value of short-term, nontraumatic stressors. Kelly McGonigal, PhD, adds engaging, informative, and empowering ideas to the mix with her book, *The Upside of Stress*, a science-based look at how you can get good at stress and why you would want to (McGonigal, 2015). Science shows us that our stress responses, or stress thresholds, are as individualized as our personalities or body types. So, managing our stress responses is a necessary part of health and wellbeing, not just good advertising. Let's look at what is called the HPA axis, the starting place for personalizing your stress response and gaining more insight into trauma. 'Be informed and be inspired'.

The HPA axis begins in the thalamus with threat detection (Figure 1.4). The thalamus sends signals to the amygdala. If danger or stress has been detected, the amygdala sends signals to the hypothalamus, which then releases the corticotropin-releasing hormone (CRH). The pituitary gland secretes the adrenocorticotropic hormone (ACTH) and so it begins. Feedback loops between the brain and body, fed by

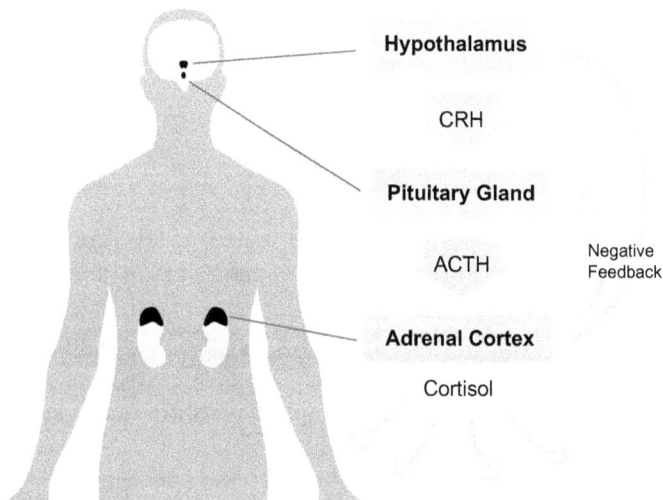

**Hypothalamus**

CRH

**Pituitary Gland**

ACTH          Negative Feedback

**Adrenal Cortex**

Cortisol

**Figure 1.4** The HPA Axis

signals of danger or safety from the thalamus, all work to get us back to homeostasis. Remember, signals can come from interoception, exteroception, and neuroception: both conscious and unconscious signals power the cycle. The termination of the stress response is critical for maintaining a healthy system. The takeaway point is there is a lot going on, not all of it fully understood, as neurotransmitters and hormones cycle through the body. The last section of this chapter looks at why breathwork and movement are tools everyone can use to personalize their stress feedback loops, which is practicing self-regulation. The workings of your HPA axis have a strong effect on the fourth part of the limbic model, the hippocampus.

4.  **Hippocampus:** The memory of an event is encoded but not stored in the hippocampus. There are two types. One type is implicit or nonverbal memory – how a preverbal child encodes a memory. Implicit memory is based on body sensation, emotional memory, motor memory, and perceptual memory. Explicit or narrative memory has words and is encoded with a time stamp: that was then, this is now (Siegel, 2020). One relevant point is stress hormone levels directly affect memory encoding. The second is that memories are not stored in the hippocampus but sent to other areas. Habits, or actions that are done without thought, are stored in the basal ganglia, cerebellum, and brainstem (subcortical). Therein lies the trauma piece to be discussed in the section on what trauma, the changes in the body and brain wrought by stress, can do to the triune brain. In the late 1800s Pierre Janet, MD, coined the term subconscious to describe how memories are automatically stored (van der Kolk, 1989). He also formulated the idea that traumatic memories are stored in ways that are different from memories of ordinary events. Research into traumatic memories is ongoing.

**The Neocortex – Let's Talk About It:** The newest part of the evolved brain, from the Latin *cortic* meaning tree bark, is unique to mammals. The neocortex is the seat of language, thought, higher-level thinking, judgement, reason, imagination, working memory, self-sensing, and empathy. Yet it takes up only 30 percent of the brain. This part of the brain allows us to think and talk about things (prefrontal cortex), to notice how we feel (insula and medial prefrontal cortex), and to consider the feelings of others (anterior insular cortex). That is, we take the time to consider possibilities, outcomes, and consequences. Of interest to anyone who interacts with teens: this part of the brain is not fully functional, fully integrated with other parts, until someone is in their midtwenties (Sapolsky, 2017). Asking a teen or someone with unresolved trauma,

"What is wrong with you?" could be answered with, "Some parts of my brain are not fully integrated."

## The Polyvagal Theory (PVT)

In 1995, Stephen Porges provided a much-needed update to the simple on/off switch or hot/cold nervous system model (Porges, 1994). His accessible discussions on vagal brakes, human imperatives, social engagement, and physiological platforms have inspired many body-based clinical and teaching applications for trauma recovery and building resiliency skills. Let's take a deeper look at what these ideas mean and their relevance to trauma work, whether personal or professional. Dr. Porges' research continues to bring clarity and focus to the trauma conversation as he explores the many layers that go into creating a sense of safety.

**The Vagus Nerve:** The vagus nerve is the 10th cranial nerve, called the pneumogastric by Charles Darwin in the late 1800s. It is the primary nerve in the parasympathetic nervous system, regulating such autonomic functions as heart rate, breathing, and digestion (Figure 1.5). Here is the really interesting piece. These vagal nerve pathways connect the brainstem areas to areas in the body that include the neck, chest, and abdomen. Therefore, your feelings of excitement, fear, or even feeling nothing at all (flat affect) are expressed in

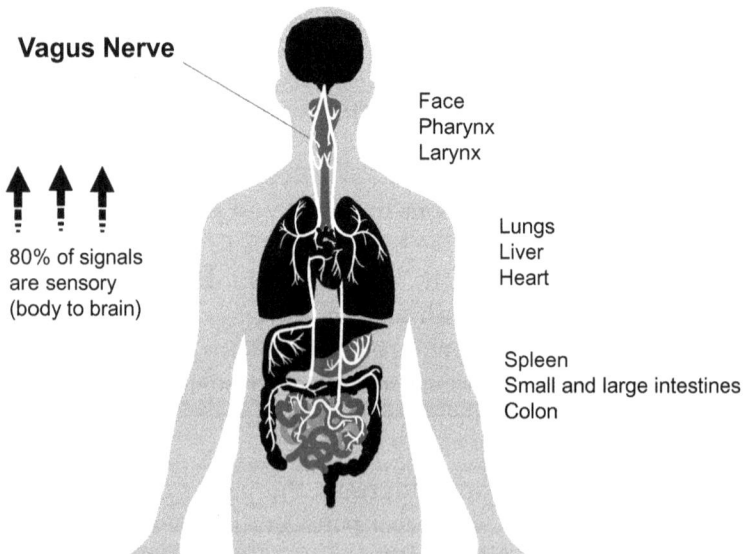

**Vagus Nerve**

80% of signals
are sensory
(body to brain)

Face
Pharynx
Larynx

Lungs
Liver
Heart

Spleen
Small and large intestines
Colon

**Figure 1.5** The Vagus Nerve

your facial expressions. There is more. Your feelings, via these neural pathways, also affect your tone of voice and how your brain processes and interprets sounds. The vagus nerve has many connections, which explains why it was named for the Latin word for wandering, *vagus*.

Again, did you notice that 80 percent of the signals run from the body to the brain? Keep that front and center in your trauma-informed mind as we look a bit more closely at the polyvagal theory. As Bessel van der Kolk notes, this vagal nerve fact gives us many possibilities for using the body for trauma recovery (van der Kolk, 2015). This fact also explains why the renowned neuroscientist Antonio Damasio, PhD, says that our sense of who we are is anchored to how we connect to our body: "A mind is so closely shaped by the body … no body, never mind" (Damasio, 1999).

**Social Engagement – System Override:** The polyvagal theory (PVT), states that mammalian responses to stimuli are organized in a three-tiered system based on evolutionary development.

Let's talk about the exciting point the PVT brings front and center in thinking about treating trauma. The freeze response (instinctive) or fight-or-flight (emotional) can be overridden in mammals by activating something Dr. Porges calls the social engagement system, the third-tier response (Porges, 2011, 2017). But how?

Emotional override, or the vagal brake, is possible because over time mammals developed faster, myelinated pathways connecting to the facial muscles, to the larynx in the throat, and to the muscles controlling the tympanic membrane (eardrum). Again, these connections are why feelings of safety can influence how we sound, our facial expressions, and how we process sound signals. There is a flip side. Consider someone calls, "Are you there?" You either respond, "Be there in a minute, I need to finish this," or you race to see what is wrong. How did you decide? If you raced to help, increased levels of stress hormones may have caused a constriction in the muscles modulating that person's voice. Or quite simply, they sounded very upset. If you had seen their face, you would have detected that facial stress. Interestingly, another piece of the trauma puzzle is someone in this stressed state may only hear low deep tones, a physiological default mode for danger detection (Porges, 2011). To some, the world can continually be perceived as a dangerous place.

**A New Kind of Imperative:** A key point in the PVT is what Dr. Porges considers a biological imperative: human connection (Porges, 2011). Why is human connection a biological imperative? Dr. Porges explains we use other humans to co-regulate, which helps us navigate our world and our feelings.

He continues with a point key to trauma recovery: instead of using our physical and emotional resources to deal with stress, co-regulating means can use those resources instead to maintain physical and mental health. You may be thinking some service animals or pets provide safety cues and points of connection. You may be thinking about a child with a caregiver, perhaps a parent with unresolved trauma, who lacks the ability to convey those cues. As a result, the child fails to develop critical self-regulation skills early in life. Or perhaps a child's caregiver was more volatile, leading the child to become hyperaware of shifts in mood signaled by facial expression or vocal cues. You may be thinking of some prison systems that are reclassifying solitary confinement as cruel and unusual punishment. Indeed, human connection as a biological imperative gives those working with trauma a lot with which to work.

On a relevant mental health note, Vivek H. Murthy, MD, Surgeon General of the United States under two presidents, wrote a book called *Together: The Healing Power of Human Connection in a Sometimes Lonely World*, in which he discusses the science of why we seek social connections. Indeed, researchers continue to show the biological imperative of connection is mediated by levels of oxytocin, dopamine, and endorphins. Being socially connected is a healthy set point because it is part of our homeostatic regulation. Or quite simply, having a friendly chat or a cup of tea with someone can make us feel better. Remember Piglet taking Pooh's paw. "I just wanted to be sure of you." Studies continue to show that social connection is a strong protective factor and supports trauma recovery and building resilience. Reviewing a growing body of scientific literature, including the many scientific works of John Cacioppo, PhD, led Dr. Murthy to conclude that "our drive to connect is one of our most important survival instincts" (Murthy, 2021).

My South African friend and a talented yoga teacher signs her emails, Ubuntu Makwande. She explained that *ubuntu* is an African principle and philosophy widely embraced by communities in South Africa. The principle seeks to express the importance of the extension of humanity (communal acts of kindness, love, care, compassion) to all beings. Or quite simply, it expresses that 'I am, because we are'. The word *makwande* is added, which means let it flourish/expand/extend to all beings. Ubuntu Makwande is a principle you may want to bring to your trauma recovery and resiliency skills program. Or it may be a phrase with which to end your emails.

**Red Light, Green Light:** Dr. Porges's use of a stoplight metaphor is instructive (Porges, 2017). In a healthy, adaptive brain, signals are clearly processed and appropriate. Does someone freeze (red light)? Does a situation demand a more immediate response of movement with fight-or-flight (green light)? Or can a pause (yellow light) allow time for the social engagement system (the vagal brake) to override the instinctive or emotional response with a more thoughtful response? What expressions show the physiological fact that signals take longer to go from the thalamus to the neocortex (thought) than from the thalamus to the amygdala (emotion)? "Just count to ten," "Give me a minute to collect my thoughts," and "Take a few deep breaths before you do anything," come to mind. It's the age-old wisdom of pausing to make the time to go from reactive to proactive. Viktor Frankl, a renowned psychiatrist and Holocaust survivor of four concentration camps is credited with saying, "Between stimulus and response there is a space. In that space is our power to choose our response. In our response lies our growth and our freedom." We will circle back to how these ideas are relevant to empowering yourself or someone else to take the time to choose a response. This empowerment involves practicing the tools of simple breathwork and movement.

**Set Up for Success:** Stephen Porges argues that the simple stimulus-response paradigm misses an important opportunity for guiding treatment. We do not all respond to the same stimulus with the same response. That is, different people, different responses. But different people, different responses is only part of it. Because someone will not always have the same response. "Usually that wouldn't bother me, but …" But what?

Dr. Porges identifies "the importance of the physiological state as an intervening variable influencing behavior and our ability to interact with others" (Porges, 2017). It's a mouthful. But the idea is worth teasing apart as it has simple and practical applications as you, personally or professionally, support trauma recovery and building resiliency skills. "I am too upset to talk about this now, so let me take a walk first." Someone is trying for a new frame of mind to guide a different response. Most of us know a physiological state, for example feeling calm or anxious, influences how we respond. The physiological state is determined in part by what neurotransmitters have been released, based on a situation – again, either real or perceived. If you are looking at someone too depressed to attend to you or someone in a blind rage, you are looking at intervening variables.

Strong science supports considering someone's physiological state as you guide rebuilding a sense of safety. Part of this consideration is how to empower someone to first recognize their feeling state and then, if they choose, take steps to change it, that is, to self-regulate. You are a part of the initial process, as you bring *your* physiological state to the game as well (see Chapter 5). "The importance of the physiological state as an intervening variable influencing behavior and our ability to interact with others" is an organizing theme of this book, so perhaps give this section another read. I know spending some time teasing it apart helped me frame the story I wanted to tell in my trainings and in this book.

## Window of Tolerance

Daniel Siegel coined the term window of tolerance to describe the degree of arousal in which a person can function without disruption (Siegel, 2020). Or how much stress can someone handle before cognitive functions are impaired? Or quite simply, how long before someone has a meltdown, blows their top, or has a come-apart? We now know that what you perceive as stressful or safe feeds your stress response and defines your personal window of tolerance. And remember all the talk of neuroplasticity and our ability to change our brains and how we are not stuck? Well, your current window of tolerance is not set in stone. It is, rather, set in your ability to rewire your brain.

That ability to change your window of tolerance is the takeaway point as you guide both yourself and others to manage stress, both real and perceived. Elizabeth Stanley, PhD, entitled her book *Widen the Window* (Stanley, 2019). It takes a deep dive into the science and some strategies for retraining your brain and body toward adaptive responses after trauma and other stresses. Peter Levine, PhD, uses the phrase islands of safety to denote that space in which someone feels safe enough to access their own tools for recovery. The idea being that through empowering someone in trauma recovery and building resiliency skills, the islands of safety can grow (Levine, 2012). He also talks about the idea of pendulation, or the ability to increase stress thresholds by moving in and out of uncomfortable sensations. How these ideas support using body-based yoga as a tool to increase stress thresholds is discussed in this chapter's last section.

**Play to Widen the Window:** Old school thinking was that play had no place in the serious business of trauma recovery. Yet yoga philosophy teaches *lila* as a quality to bring to your practice, a quality of play or sport engaged in without self-consciousness or limitations imposed by distractions of specific outcomes. Or quite simply, "Hey, try something new – what have you got to lose?" Okay, but why is play discussed in the science section of this book? Because it turns out scientists study what play does to the brain (Panksepp, 2011). Playing, in both children and adults, stimulates the brainstem area called the periaqueductal grey (PAG), which secretes endogenous (natural) opioids. One appeal of opioids is thought to be they create feelings of safety. Feeling safe allows time for the prefrontal cortex to explore different scenarios and to become more plastic, more able to rewire (Huberman, 2022). So, if a key part of trauma recovery is, as Bessel van der Kolk teaches us, becoming curious and imagining different outcomes, and if a body-based yoga practice can support that sense of play, then the science of play becomes quite exciting to consider (van der Kolk, 2015). Stephen Porges writes that play provides opportunities to experience a disruption of the autonomic state (you get anxious or unsure), a feeling which is then stabilized using the social engagement system (you self-regulate by attuning to other mammals) (Porges, 2021). Bringing a sense of play to your teaching or your personal yoga practice means you have another tool to support rewiring neural pathways and to widen windows tolerance. Before you teach in movie-themed costumes or with silly games, perhaps consider reading the rest of this book. A trauma-informed guide continues to be: 'More is not better, more is confusing'.

Let's consider what happened to narrow someone's window of tolerance, to shrink their island of safety, or to lose their ability to play before we continue with using the GreenTREE Yoga® Approach to support these neuroplastic changes, Let's look at how trauma impacts a sense of safety.

## What Does Trauma Do to That Sense of Safety?

### Mixed Signals

How do the brain signals become so muddled and conflicting that someone does not pause to think (yellow light) but always responds with a full red or green light? How does a window of tolerance narrow so that someone's life lacks joy because everything is stressful? Let's consider that the damage caused by the physiological stresses of trauma starts at the cellular level. Again, our brain has over 90 billion neurons. All together, these neurons are over 200 million miles long. As a fun point of reference, the Earth is about 93 million miles (150 million kilometers) from the Sun. Individually, each neuron has an average of 10,000 synapses, which create hundreds of trillions of neuronal connections.

**Your Neurons on Trauma:** Traumatic Brain Injury (TBI) is one type of damage to the brain, a physical injury to tissue that disrupts how signals are sent and processed throughout the brain and body. Another type of disruption in brain function is caused as neurotransmitters or stress hormones (among them, cortisol, adrenaline, and norepinephrine) flood the body during and after trauma. Daniel Siegel explains four ways these physiological changes can disrupt or damage cellular function (NICABM #3). Taking a deeper dive into the neuroscience can guide your program design. 'Be informed and be inspired'.

- **Neurons:** Trauma can cause neuronal death (apoptosis).
- **Synapses:** High levels of stress hormones can damage the synaptic connections as dendrites atrophy. You may be thinking – missed signals, which is exactly what happens.

- **Myelin Sheath:** The myelin sheath can be damaged over time, which slows signals. As an example, when the body's immune system attacks the myelin sheaths, scars form that block signal transmissions and cause loss of function. This painful autoimmune disease is multiple sclerosis (MS).
- **Epigenetics:** The field of epigenetics has shown that trauma affects the molecules that control gene expression, the histone and methyl groups on the outside of the gene (epigenetic). Though the DNA sequence in the gene does not change, epigenetic changes (on/off switches for expression) can be passed to the next generation. One of the most cited papers is from the lab of Michael Meaney, PhD. It shows that stressed rats gave birth to rat pups with low thresholds for stress, and the opposite was observed as well. Mothers that had not been stressed had pups with a much higher resistance to stress (Weaver et al., 2004). Much research has followed, linking the epigenetic effects to growth factors (BDNF) and hormone systems (Meany and Szyf, 2005). For more science on the effects of parental and childhood stress,. Robert Sapolsky, PhD, devotes chapters to the discussion in *Behave: The Biology of Humans at Our Best and Worst* (2018).

**A Well-timed Pause:** Perhaps you are thinking, "Hmmm, someone is not in conscious control of these cellular or physiological changes from trauma." You would be right. To review, as Dr. John Ratey says, "It takes guilt out of the equation when you recognize that there's a biological basis for certain emotional issues" (Ratey, 2007, 2012). Of course, so as not to sink into the mire of excuses, the next recovery step is for an individual to move toward reestablishing adaptive brain function and toward building personal resiliency skills. I saw a license plate on a big truck that said, "PTSD." It gave me pause as I looked at the driver, wondering if it were a warning or an excuse. As Dr. Ratey continues, "On the other hand, you won't be left feeling helpless when you see how you can influence that biology." Indeed, the excuse of, "Oh, that's just the way he is, he's not ever going to change," is not true for most people. Current science keeps the nature/nurture discussions lively.

## Connections Lost

If your building blocks or bricks are damaged, your structure will be flawed. Let's take a quick look at how damaged neurons, our personalized building blocks, impair three areas of brain function.

**The Hippocampus**, located in the limbic structure, is the place in which memories are processed and then relayed for storage in other parts of the brain. The flood of stress hormones can shrink the hippocampus due to cell death, which can affect learning. Another change is how memories initially are encoded, which we discuss in the next section. Scientists have found some lost functions can be restored (Conrad, 2008). Again, we are not stuck.

**The Corpus Callosum** is a thick, fibrous bundle of nerve fibers that connects the right-brain/left-brain hemispheres, a conduit for motor, sensory, and cognitive information. Damage to these transmission pathways causes slower or missed signals.

**The Neocortex** is key in both the up–down integration of other brain structures and in integrating parts within the prefrontal cortex. Damage to these neuronal connections can affect how the thinking (the prefrontal cortex), emotion (the limbic system), and instinctive responses (the reptilian brain) coordinate and integrate functions.

## The Triune Brain Revisited

Many book titles put the body front and center in trauma discussions. *When the Body Says No* (Maté, 2011), *The Body Keeps the Score* (van der Kolk, 2015), *Trauma and the Body* (Ogden, 2006), *The Body Remembers* (Rothchild, 2000), and *In an Unspoken Voice: How the Body Releases Trauma and Restores Goodness* (Levine, 2010) are but a few examples. Taking a cue from many trauma experts, let's consider the body and trauma disruptions.

**Basic Body Functions:** Trauma stored in the body can present as sleep disorders, sexual dysfunction, flashbacks, and many types of digestive or eating disorders. You may be saying, "What does that mean, 'stored in the body'?" That is indeed the question to ask. One trauma piece is stress levels affect how the memories are first encoded in the hippocampus. Increased levels of cortisol interfere with the formation of explicit memories, stored as words in the neocortex as part of a narrative with a time stamp. It's a way to make sense of what happens. Interestingly, many scientists believe that this final processing occurs during REM sleep. Unprocessed memory fragments can disrupt many bodily functions.

There is more. Increased levels of another stress hormone, epinephrine (adrenaline) increase the encoding of implicit, or nonverbal, memories. These nonverbal memories then are stored in the reptilian or survival brain or the brainstem, specifically in the basal ganglia. With no story line and no time stamp, these memories are recorded as body sensations, a perceptual memory of the event, or a flashback (Siegel, 2012). That implicit memory encoding is one way trauma is stored in the body. An insightful book for your trauma library is *Trauma and Memory: Brain and Body in a Search for the Living Past* by Peter Levine (2015). Vincent J. Felitti, MD, one of the researchers in the ACES (Adverse Child Experiences) study, identified childhood traumas as predictive of many health issues later in life. He explained that his interest grew as he noted many of his patients with obesity issues had experienced childhood traumas (Felitti et al., 1998).

**Getting Stuck in Overdrive:** What does disruption from trauma look like in the limbic system? As Besel van der Kolk explains, trauma causes the threat detection system to malfunction. With everything perceived as danger, someone can get stuck in a state of hypervigilance. Being stuck means the HPA axis keeps going, with no vagal brake and no decrease in stress hormones. Again, short-term stress stimulates our immune function. But, over time, the body may begin to attack its own tissues (Stanley, 2019). Purely anecdotally, I noticed that almost all (yes, almost all) of the veterans with PTSD diagnoses I worked with over ten years had one or more autoimmune issues.

**No Time to Talk:** Results of trauma also play out in the neocortex, with direct implications for trauma recovery protocols. We have discussed that feelings of fear or rage override the neocortex function (thought) with faster-acting emotion or survival instincts. What expressions illustrate emotional hijacking? "I feel like my head is going to explode," and "I can't think straight," come to mind. This understanding of body physiology has been expressed in our everyday language long before brain scans and biomarker stress tests.

Another result of trauma is that because of faulty memory encoding, someone may in fact not be able to access implicit memories with words. They may not be trying to be difficult or resistant. They truly cannot find the words because they are not there to be found. This fact is why such trauma experts as Pat Ogden, Peter Levine, and Bessel van der Kolk say that someone does not have to first tell their story. Therapists can begin resolving trauma with body-based modalities.

Trauma also can cause diminished function in the dorsolateral prefrontal cortex, the time-keeper in the brain. This fact is part of why trauma can cause someone to get stuck in the past. Over time stronger neuronal connections are created as someone continues to relive the event fragment not attached to any narrative giving it a time stamp. "Trauma is a disease of not being able to be present ..." as Pierre Janet, MD, wrote in the late 1880s (van der Kolk, 2015). Two other parts of the prefrontal cortex with greatly diminished activation are the insula and the medial prefrontal cortex, the places of self-sensing and of emotional and physical awareness. This science leads us directly to what a body-based yoga practice brings to this important discussion.

## Why Are Breath and Movement the Safety Net?

### The Ebb and the Flow: Heart Rate Variability

Heart Rate Variability (HRV) is our most central natural rhythm, the way in which how we breathe can influence our heart rate. Why is the fact that breathing affects heart rate an exciting notion in our trauma discussion? Because it means that with conscious effort, we can manage how we breathe. If we practice how we breathe, we can manage our heart rate, blood pressure, and therefore our stress response. It means we can personalize our stress cycle. Let's consider the fascinating science of breathing.

Let's go back to the term homeostasis to clarify the connection between breath and heart rate. From the Greek words *homoios* and *stasis*, it means to stay the same. Homeostasis refers to physiological processes that maintain conditions necessary for survival. It's like the 'Middle Way' for the body, or a life-affirming process to come back from physiological extremes. The

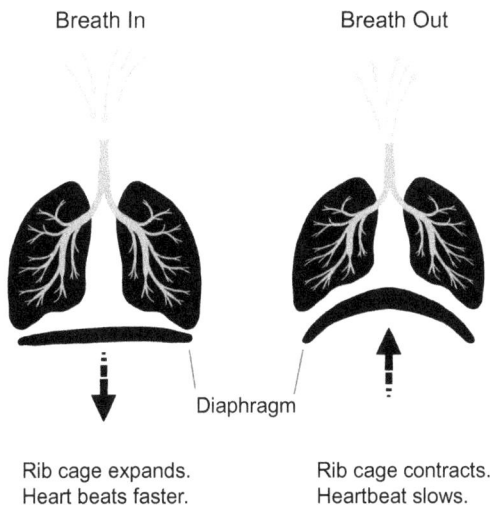

Breath In                    Breath Out

Diaphragm

Rib cage expands.          Rib cage contracts.
Heart beats faster.        Heartbeat slows.

**Figure 1.6** The Diaphragm: Major Muscle of Respiration

science of breathing gives insight into these homeostatic mechanisms in action.

The diaphragm is a dome-shaped muscle that stretches across the bottom of the rib cage (Figure 1.6). This muscle is innervated by the autonomic nervous system, that is it moves as we breathe without us having to think about it. Imagine if we had to think about each and every 20,000 or so breaths we take in a day. Here is an interesting note for practicing self-regulation tools. We can consciously move this diaphragm muscle when we decide to practice a deep breath in or a deep breath out. Understanding this process can empower you to be more effective both in your professional work and at providing self-care. As I teach in my workshops, self-care is not being selfish, it's being practical.

You could read about it. Or perhaps, in the spirit of experiential learning, give yourself a few moments and try the following. When you are ready, look at the left side of Figure 1.6 and practice a long breath in. Keep practicing longer breaths in, if that is comfortable for you today. Envision your lungs expanding. The negative pressure created by the dropping of the dome-shaped diaphragm is what expands the lungs. If you continue with longer breaths in, you may begin to feel faint. However, your body naturally tends toward homeostasis, so envision that with those longer breaths in, a signal is being sent via the vagus nerve from the sinoatrial (SA) node in your heart to your brainstem. The signal is your heart rate is slowing, which is causing your blood pressure to drop. In a healthy system that tends toward homeostasis, a new signal now is being sent from your brainstem back to your heart. Now your heart beats faster and harder, to maintain the blood pressure you need to respond to the current situation. That fact is why longer breaths in can be energizing, getting you ready for action. Again, it is your body self-regulating.

Okay, so what does a longer breath out do? To experience this part of breath science in real-time, look at the right side of Figure 1.6. As you are ready, feel your breath in. Then practice a longer breath out as you envision your diaphragm muscle releasing, like a rubber band returning to its at-rest shape. No active energy is being used by that dome-shaped muscle. Keep practicing longer, slow breaths out if that is comfortable for you today. The signals being sent via your vagus nerve from the SA node in your heart to the brainstem have changed. The new signals are that your system does not need as much oxygen. So your heart rate slows, then your blood pressure decreases.

How did you manage your heart rate and blood pressure and stress response? Again, your body automatically tends toward homeostasis, which can happen with a few breath cycles. The answer is you achieved control by managing how you breathe. Exciting stuff. It should be noted that for those with heart or lung disease, breathwork can be an effective additional treatment modality to be explored after seeking proper medical consultation. Also note that for some, either of these breathing patterns can be agitating. More on this idea in the chapters on the breath.

## Movement

Joseph LeDoux, PhD, introduced the idea of defensive survival circuits. His research showed that fear signals can be redirected from the central nucleus in the amygdala, which can cause irrational fears, to the basal nucleus that connects to the body's motor pathways. "By engaging these alternative pathways, the passive fear response is replaced with an effective coping strategy" (LeDoux, 2015). This redirection can occur from action or from thought. Accessing these alternate pathways has been practiced for thousands of years by many cultures, calming the nervous system with breath, movement, and rhythm. Let's also note that moving in a group, perhaps dancing, singing, or chanting, has the benefit of activating the social engagement system. Many forms of prayer involve chanting and rocking as well. Again, moving our bodies is fundamental to how we self-regulate, moving away from danger or moving toward safety (van der Kolk, 2015; Porges, 2011). Current science supports thousands of years of empirical data from across cultures, data gathered from both observation and experience.

Such neurotransmitters as serotonin, norepinephrine, and dopamine are released when we move. We know that many pharmacological treatments (medications) for anxiety and depression are designed to regulate and manipulate levels of these key neurotransmitters. Selective serotonin reuptake inhibitors (SSRIs) and ketamine are examples.

But there is so much more to the story. Research has shown the levels of glutamate and GAMA are increased as we move (Maddock, 2016). The reason that many drugs work is that our body creates some forms naturally, so we already have the receptors. Opioids are an example. Runner's high happens when our bodies release such endogenous (natural) opioids as endorphins and endocannabinoids, both of which inhibit pain and improve mood. Research continues to show that acetylcholine levels increase with movement, specifically in the hippocampus and cortex. These changes support the neuroplastic changes of stronger synaptic connections and memory formations. Or quite simply, moving can improve the ability to learn (Giocomo, 2007).

Not done yet. Movement also supports cellular repair processes, as described by the Harvard evolutionary biologist Daniel E. Lieberman, PhD, in *Exercised: Why Something We Never Evolved to Do Is Healthy and Rewarding* (2020). The book presents current studies and ideas on the benefits of exercise and serves as a strong complement to John Ratey's foundational book, *Spark: The Revolutionary New Science of Exercise and the Brain* (2008/2013). When we move, changes in brain chemistry improve brain structure and create healthier neurons. Our bodies also make many types of growth factors. Of particular interest to our trauma discussion is brain-derived neurotrophic factor (BDNF). Levels of BDNF increase during exercise and are key to repairing neurons (Saucedo-Marquez et al., 2015; Basso et al., 2017). As John Ratey explains in much detail in *Spark*, exercise inoculates the brain against stress because it increases growth factors (Ratey, 2008/2013). Movement, then, helps to build resiliency skills as it increases our stress thresholds. In addition, studies have shown that when we move, a hormone called atrial natriuretic peptide (ANP) is released from the heart tissue – the faster the heart beats, the more is released. This molecule interrupts the HPA cycle. Studies show that ANP plays a role in the neurobiology of anxiety (Koopman, 2014). Regular exercise also lowers cortisol levels (Duclos, 2016). Moving also increases the blood supply to the brain, which can improve brain health and memory function (Raichlen, 2017).

Research and discovery are ongoing as to the specific benefits of different exercises. Yet the overall message is resoundingly clear. Movement promotes a healthier body and a healthier brain, starting at the cellular level and building from there. In addition, movements that involve something novel or complex (think new yoga poses) increase and strengthen different neural networks (Basso et al., 2017; Ratey, 2013). The words of John Ratey speak directly to trauma recovery:

> The stress of exercise is predictable and controllable because you're Initiating the action … With exercise, you gain a sense of mastery and self-confidence. As you develop awareness of your own ability to manage stress and not rely on negative coping mechanism, you increase your ability to 'snap out of it' … you learn to trust that you can deal with it.
>
> (Ratey, 2013)

Understanding that we have ever-changing brains based on the interplay of brain, body, and the environment, Pat Ogden a renowned trauma therapist, advises in her foundational book, *Trauma and the Body* (2006), that we can use the body to restructure cognition. But of course, only if the signals are working. Now we need to put it all together.

## Putting It All Together: Getting Unstuck with Yoga

Let's identify some scientific reasons that yoga, a body-based modality for connecting mind and body using the breath, can be a trauma recovery tool and can build resiliency skills. How can yoga support what Daniel Siegel calls regulation through integration, by which he means facilitating the reintegration of different parts of the brain that trauma may have damaged? (Siegel, 2012/2020). How does yoga support Pat Ogden's advice to use the body as the entry point to the emotions? (Ogden, 2007). How does yoga support Ron Siegel's variation on Freud's idea of using dreams as the royal road to the unconscious to using the body is the royal road to the unconscious? (NICABM #1). How can yoga do what B.S.K. Iyengar said in *Light on Life*: "Yoga allows you to rediscover a sense of wholeness in your life, where you do not feel like you are constantly trying to fit broken pieces together" (Iyengar, 1966/1976). An informative look at yoga philosophy as it relates to trauma, outside of the scope of this book, is in *Yoga for Trauma Recovery* by Lisa Danylchuk (2010).

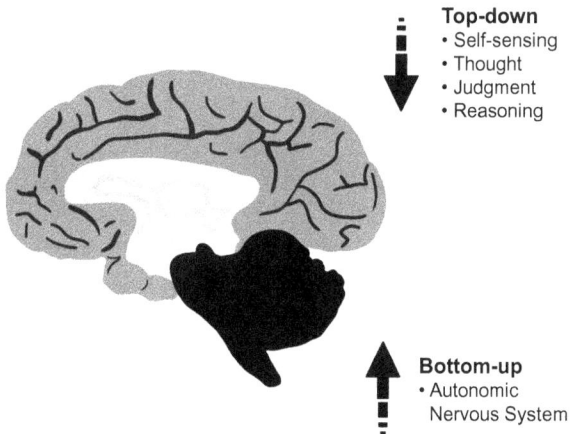

**Top-down**
• Self-sensing
• Thought
• Judgment
• Reasoning

**Bottom-up**
• Autonomic
  Nervous System

**Figure 1.7** Top-Down and Bottom-Up

**Getting Clear Directions:** We can say that yoga puts it all together because it is both top-down and bottom-up. Top-down means yoga activates the self-sensing parts of the brain. Bottom-up means yoga can help someone to manage their autonomic nervous system. Or quite simply, it can help someone to self-regulate. As discussed, it is sensory input (bottom-up) that powers our instinctive or emotional responses.

**Top-down:** As discussed, top-down refers to self-sensing or the awareness of how we feel. Is being able to recognize a feeling of stress or discomfort or pleasure important in trauma recovery? Bessel van der Kolk tells us:

> Traumatized people chronically feel unsafe inside their bodies: The past is alive in the form of gnawing interior discomfort. Their bodies are constantly bombarded by visceral warning signs, and, in an attempt to control these processes, they often become expert at ignoring their gut feelings and in numbing awareness of what is played out inside. They learn to hide from their selves.
>
> (van der Kolk, 2015)

Hiding feelings from yourself or numbing can mean the self-sensing parts of the brain are not functioning well. Moshe Feldenkrais' insight highlights the issue: "You can't do what you want until you know what you are doing" (van der Kolk, 2015). Peer-reviewed studies have shown that yoga can reactivate the insula and medial prefrontal cortex, the self-sensing parts of the cortex. Interestingly, these cortical areas are located behind the sixth chakra called the third eye, the seat of awareness, perception, and intuition in yoga philosophy.

**Bottom-up:** Bottom-up refers to how the body relays sensory signals to the brain. Brain scans of the homunculus (brain maps of the body) show the areas of the hands, lips, and feet as cartoonishly large because of the high concentrations of sense receptors. As one example, we have four main types of mechanoreceptors: Merkel cells, Meissner cells, Pacinian corpuscles, and Ruffini nerve fibers. These cells pick up different sensory information – pressure, tapping, and high- or low-frequency vibrations. This science is particularly useful to yoga teachers in planning ways to help people build self-awareness. Consider that high concentrations of receptors in the feet help us to gather information, both conscious and reflexive, to stand, move, and balance (Strzalkowski, 2018). So it makes sense that top-down and bottom-up connections can be strengthened with breathwork and movement. It comes back to how the neurons function, which is why this chapter started with the basics on neurons and how the brain can change.

**Vagus Nerve Revisited:** To review, 80 percent of the vagal nerve fibers are sensory and run from the body to the brain. This fact means many opportunities exist to use the body (bottom-up) to calm the nervous system, as Bessel van der Kolk notes, adding, "Insight does not quiet the limbic system" (NICABM #3, 2014). Talking about something (top-down) will not calm someone not fully using the verbal part of the brain (van der Kolk, 2015). Let's not wander too far from the breath in the trauma conversation. Stephen Porges explains that breathing gates the influence of the vagus nerve on the heart. Longer breaths in decrease the influence of the vagus nerve, so heart rate increases. And the opposite is true. Longer breaths out can slow the heart rate. With good heart rate variability (HRV), someone is not stuck with a heart rate that is always racing or always very slow.

A yoga practice, which is both breathwork and movement, can improve heart rate variability (van der Kolk, 2014). As we do yoga, the heart rate can speed up during more challenging poses and then slow down during more restful poses. Again, a central yoga principle is balancing steadiness (*sthira*) and ease (*sukha*). It makes sense that teaching in a way that balances effort and ease can be key in creating opportunities for someone to experience not being stuck. The practice sequences in Chapter 11 create many of these experiential opportunities.

**Top-down/Bottom-up:** While doing a warrior two flow, someone may feel their heart rate increase with the effort. Then, guided by a trauma-informed teacher, they may notice they can, quite literally, breathe and move through the stress. Someone can experience in real-time the rhythm of their breathing and heart beating, the rhythm of speeding up and slowing down, all within the safety of a trauma-informed setting. This key point in trauma recovery and building resiliency skills bears repeating. Someone chooses to move in and out of warrior two – feeling discomfort, literally moving through it, and noticing that they are still okay. These feelings and thoughts may be processed at both cortical (thinking) and subcortical (emotional/instinctive) levels. "Felt some discomfort, kept moving, still breathing, listening to my instructor's voice, coming out when I want." Some may not use words but simply *feel* some discomfort or stress. Then, they find an alternate way of processing and responding using the tools of breath and movement. Yoga sets the stage for two keys in trauma recovery, as noted by. Bessel van der Kolk: notice that and what happens next (van der Kolk, 2015). Noticing means sensing something, and then processing those feelings in the present. Becoming curious about what happens next helps rebuild a sense of time. Top-down, bottom-up.

**Mindfulness:** The GreenTREE Yoga® Approach teaches body-based yoga, one that connects the mind and body using the breath. So where does that put mindfulness and meditation in our discussion? As John Kabat-Zinn, PhD, says, "Mindfulness means paying attention in a particular way: on purpose, in the present moment, and non-judgmentally"(Kabat-Zinn, 1994). For someone with a narrow window of tolerance at the beginning of trauma recovery, sitting or lying down without body movements to help ground, whether in a meditation or mindfulness practice, can miss the mark. Dr. Kabat-Zinn puts a finer point on it in his comment to Bessel van der Kolk: "I think it is malpractice to practice meditation without doing yoga for people with trauma" (NICABM #2).

In *Widen the Window*, Elizabeth Stanley, PhD, offers that meditation or mindfulness practices may in fact make someone's dysregulation worse, becoming more aware of their dysregulated state without the tools to self-regulate (Stanley, 2019). As Bessel van der Kolk notes, "Yoga organizes your attentional system into very specific movements and postures and keeps you away from the free-floating residue that comes up when you do meditation" (NICABM, #2). We will come back to this key idea. Both Peter Levine and Pat Ogden provide trauma trainings using somatic resources. Bessel van der Kolk devotes an entire chapter to yoga in his best-selling book, *The Body Keeps the Score*. The rest of this book explains how the science-based GreenTREE Yoga® Approach can empower someone to manage their breath, their body, and their responses.

**********

**To Recap:** This chapter introduces several key points that frame the GreenTREE Yoga® Approach for building safety, supporting empowerment, and maintaining simplicity. The brain's ability to rewire in a more adaptive way can continue throughout the lifespan. We need to continually remind ourselves that if someone does not feel safe, they cannot learn new things and may be stuck in maladaptive defensive strategies. It also is important to keep in our trauma-informed minds that this physiological state often is not under conscious control.

So, should we care about how the brain works? It merits repeating John Ratey's words:

> Your life changes when you have a working knowledge of your brain. It takes guilt out of the equation when you recognize that there's a biological basis for certain emotional issues. On the other hand, you won't be left feeling helpless when you see how you can influence that biology.
>
> (Ratey, 2008/2013)

You may now, after considering some neuroscience, have a better understanding of the answer to the question posed at the beginning: "Are we stuck?" Based on body physiology and the brain's ability to change, we are not stuck. We each can develop and regain the tools to create lives that can allow us what Victor Frankl, a psychiatrist and survivor of four concentration camps, called "The last of the human freedoms: to choose one's attitude in any given set of circumstances, to choose one's own way." ~ Viktor Frankl in *Man's Search for Meaning*

## References

Basso, Julia C., et al. (2017). The Effects of Acute Exercise on Mood, Cognition, Neurophysiology, and Neurochemical Pathways: A Review. *Brain Plasticity*, 2(2), 127–152.

Butts, Daniel A., et al. (2007). A Burst-Based "Hebbian" Learning Rule at Retinogeniculate Synapses Links Retinal Waves to Activity-Dependent Refinement. *PLoS Biology*, 5(3), e61. doi: 10.1371/journal.pbio.0050061.

Cannon, Walter B. (1929). *Bodily Changes in Pain, Hunger, Fear, and Rage*. New York: Appleton, Century, Crofts.

Conrad, Cheryl D. (2008). Chronic Stress-Induced Hippocampal Vulnerability: The Glucocorticoid Vulnerability Hypothesis. *Reviews in the Neurosciences*, 19(6), 395–412.

Damasio, Antonio. (1999). *The Feeling of What Happens: Body and Emotions in the Making of Consciousness*. New York: Harcourt, p. 142.

Danylchuk, Lisa. (2019). *Yoga for Trauma Recovery: Theory, Philosophy, and Practice*. New York: Routledge Press.

Doidge, Norman. (2007). *The Brain That Changes Itself: Stories of Personal Triumph from the Frontiers of Brain Science*. New York: Viking Books.

Doidge, Norman. (2016). *The Brain's Way of Healing: Remarkable Discoveries and Recoveries from the Frontiers of Neuroplasticity*. New York: Penguin Life.

Doré, Bruce P., et al. (2017). Helping Others Regulate Emotion Predicts Increased Regulation of One's Own Emotions and Decreased Symptoms of Depression. *Personality and Social Psychology Bulletin*, 43(5), 729–739.

Jinek, M., Chylinski, K., Fonfara, I., Hauer, M., Doudna, J.A., Charpentier, E. (2012). A Programmable Dual-RNA-Guided DNA Endonuclease in Adaptive Bacterial Immunity. Science, 337(6096), 816–821.

Duclos, Martine. (2016). Exercise and the HPA Axis. *Frontiers in Hormone Research*, 47, 12–26.

Eagleman, David. (2020). *Livewired: The Inside Story of the Everchanging Brain*. New York: Vintage.

Felliti, Vincent J., et al. (1998). The Relationship of Adult Health Status to Childhood Abuse and Household Dysfunction. *American Journal of Preventive Medicine*, 14, 245–258.

Giocomo, L. M. and Hasselmo, M. E. (2007). Neuromodulation by Glutamate and Acetylcholine Can Change Circuit Dynamics by Regulating the Relative Influence of Afferent Input and Excitatory Feedback. *Molecular Neurobiology*, 36(2), 184–200.

Haase, L., et al. (2016). When the Brain Does Not Feel the Body. *Frontiers in Human Neuroscience*, 8, 770.

Haywood, E., et al. (2021). Trauma-Sensitive Yoga for Post-Traumatic Stress Disorder in Women Veterans who Experienced Military Sexual Trauma. *Journal of Alternative and Complementary Medicine*, 27(S1), S45–S59.

Hebb, Donald. (1949). *The Organization of Behaviour*. New York: John Wiley and Sons.

Huberman, Andrew. (2020–21). www.hubermanlab.com. *How Your Brain Works and Changes*. 1/1/20; *Tools for Managing Stress and Anxiety*. 3/8/21.

Iyengar, B. K. S. (1966/1976). *Light on Yoga*. Schocken Books.

James, William. (1907/1987). Pragmatism. In *William James: Writings 1902–1910*, ed. Bruce Kuklick. New York: Library of America.

Kabat-Zinn, John. (1994). *Wherever You Go, There You Are*. New York. MJF Books, p. 4.

Kandel, Eric. (2007). *In Search of Memory*. New York: W.W. Norton, p. 276.

Kelly, U., et al. (2021). Trauma-Sensitive Yoga for Post-Traumatic Stress Disorder in Women Veterans who Experienced Military Sexual Trauma. *The Journal of Alternative and Complementary Medicine*, 27(Supplement 1), S45–S59.

Koopmann, Anne, et al. (2014). The Impact of Atrial Natriuretic Peptide on Anxiety, Stress and Craving in Patients with Alcohol Dependence. *Alcohol and Alcoholism*, 49(3), 282–286.

Ledoux, Joseph. (2015). *Anxious: Using the Brain to Understand and Treat Fear and Anxiety*. New York: Viking, pp. 31–35; 211.

Levine, Peter. (1997). *Waking the Tiger: Healing Trauma*. Berkeley: North Atlantic Books, p. 87.

Levine, Peter. (2010). *In an Unspoken Voice: How the Body Releases Trauma and Restores Goodness*. Berkeley: North Atlantic Books, pp. 78–79.

Lieberman, Daniel E. (2021). *Exercised: The Science of Physical Activity, Rest and Health*. New York: Penguin.

Lucassen, Paul J., et al. (2014). Neuropathology of Stress. *Acta Neuropathologica*, 127(1), 109–135.

MacLean, Paul. (1990). *The Triune Brain in Evolution*. New York: Springer.

Maddock, R. J. et al. (2016). Acute Modulation of Cortical Glutamate and GABA by Physical Activity. *Journal of Neuroscience*, 36, 2449–2457.

Meaney, M. J. and Szyf, M. (2005). Environmental Programming of Stress Responses Through DNA Methylation. *Dialogues in Clinical Neuroscience*, 7(2), 103–123.

McGonigal, Kelly. (2016). *The Upside of Stress*. New York: Avery.

Murthy, Vivek H. (2021/2023). *Together: The Healing Power of Human Connection in a Sometimes Lonely World*. New York: Harper Paperbacks, pp. 50–51.

NICABM #1. *A TalkBack Session: Why a Body-Oriented Approach is Key for Treating Trauma with Ron Siegel, PsyD*.

NICABM #2. *When Mindfulness Will (and Won't) Work for Treating Trauma with Bessel van der Kolk, MD*.

NICABM #3. *Rethinking Trauma with Daniel Siegel, MD* (2014).

NICABM #3. *A Guide with Bessel van der Kolk, MD* (2014).

Ogden, Pat. (2006). *Trauma and the Body: A Sensorimotor Approach to Psychotherapy*. New York: W. W. Norton and Company, pp. 146; 238.

Price, Maggi, van de Kolk, Bessel A., et al. (2017). Effectiveness of an Extended Yoga Treatment for Women with Chronic PTSD. *The Journal of Alternative and Complementary Medicine*, 10(10), 1–9.

Porges, Stephen. (2011). *The Polyvagal Theory: Neurophysiological Foundations of Emotions, Attachment, Communication, and Self-regulation*. New York: W. W. Norton and Company, pp. 78–80; 87; 91; 193–194.

Porges, Stephen. (2017). *The Pocket Guide to the Polyvagal Theory: The Transformative Power of Feeling Safe*. New York: W. W. Norton and Company, pp. 21; 43; 78; 93; 108–109; 121; 191–192; 254.

Porges, Stephen. (2021). *Polyvagal Safety: Attachment, Communication, Self-Regulation (IPNB)*. New York: W. W. Norton and Company, pp. 261; 263–265.

Ratey, John. (2007/2013). *Spark: The Revolutionary New Science of Exercise and the Brain*. New York: Little, Brown, pp. 6; 104.

Sapolsky, Robert. (2018). *Behave: The Biology of Humans at Our Best and Worst*. New York: Penguin Books.

Saucedo-Marquez, C. M., et al. (2015). High-Intensity Interval Trainings Evoke Larger BDNF Levels. *Journal of Applied Physiology*, 119, 1363–1373.

Seyle, Hans. (1956/1978). *The Stress of Life*. New York: McGraw Hill.

Shatz, Carla J. (1992). The Developing Brain. *Scientific American*, 267, 60–67.

Siegel, Daniel. (2010). *Mindsight: The New Science of Personal Transformation*, 3rd edition. New York: Guildford Press and Bantam Books, pp. 18; 39–40; 155.

Siegel, Daniel. (2012). *Pocket Guide to Interpersonal Neurobiology*. New York: W. W. Norton and Company. pp. 7–2; 7–4; 7–5; 39–43.

Siegel, Daniel. (2020). *The Developing Mind: How Relationships and the Brain Interact to Shape Who We Are*, 3rd edition. New York: Guildford Press, pp. 161; 162; 316.

Siviy, Stephen and Panksepp, Jaak. (2011). In Search of the Neurobiological Substrates for Social Playfulness in Mammalian Brains. *Neuroscience and Biobehavioral Reviews*, 35(9), 1821–1830.

Stanley, Elizabeth. (2019). *Widen the Window: Training Your Brain and Body to Thrive During Stress and Recover from Trauma*. New York: Avery Publishing, p. 315.

Van der Kolk, Bessel A. (2015). *The Body Keeps the Score: Brain, Mind, and Body in the Healing of Trauma*. New York: Penguin Publishing, pp. 20–22; 92; 207–208; 210; 247; 264; 273; 349.

Van der Kolk, Bessel A., et al. (1989). Janet Pierre Janet and the Breakdown of Adaptation in Psychological Trauma. *American Journal of Psychiatry*, 146(12), 1530–1540.

Van der Kolk, Bessel A., et al. (2014). Yoga as an Adjunctive Treatment for PTSD. *The Journal of Clinical Psychiatry*, 75(6), 559–565.

Weaver, Ian, et al. (2004). Epigenetic Programming by Maternal Behavior. *Nature Neuroscience*, 7, 847–854.

Yehuda, Rachel, et al. (2014). Influences of Maternal and Paternal PTSD on Epigenetic Regulation of the Glucocorticoid Receptor Gene in Holocaust Survivor Offspring. *The American Journal of Psychiatry*, 171(8), 872–880.

Zimmer, Carl. (2023). Brain Atlas Maps 3,300 Mystery Cells. *The New York Times*. 10/15, 23.

# PART I
# Preparing to Teach

# 2
# Language

Language is a tool. In trauma recovery and in building resiliency skills that tool can build safety, support empowerment, and maintain simplicity. These three ideas create a strong synergy that may inspire you to consider the many ways in which your use of language matters. This chapter presents a general overview of trauma-informed language concepts. You will find these ideas discussed with relevant examples throughout the book. Be mindful that someone who has experienced trauma or is highly stressed may not be processing information well in the language parts of their brain. Instead, responses may come from the basic survival and emotion (subcortical) parts of the brain. Given that physiological fact, let's consider how language can help, not hinder. How do we use simple language, breathwork, and movement to get from Emily Dickinson's poetic words of "I felt a funeral in my brain …" to "I dwell in possibilities …" (Franklin, 1999)?

We know that language has different features. One is the words. Words have specific meanings, but words also carry connotations and nuances. The prosody of speech (the tone, modulation, and rhythm) is another feature. Body language conveyed through body postures and facial expressions is included as well. We will circle back to these key safety ideas. Now let's focus on the spoken word. A quote attributed to Maya Angelou comes to mind: "I've learned that people will forget what you said, people will forget what you did, but people will never forget how you made them feel." Most of us have experienced clearly remembering the *feeling* of something. Consider that the remembered feeling may have been created in part or even entirely by someone's word choice and tone of voice. A recreational therapist who attended my VA class sent a follow-up email.

> I love what you did to meet the needs of the women who were in the room. There is no need to do specific poses when it won't serve the people in the room! I loved the way you phrased things and created such

DOI: 10.4324/9781003308836-4

openness and support for wherever the women were in that moment. I remember at one point you mentioned that women could step out of a pose and said they are never stuck. Such a nice way to tie metaphor of life experiences into the practice.

**My Words to You:** People tell me they remember phrases I have developed to underscore my trauma-informed points. The following phrases in 'single quotes' throughout the book are gentle reminders of the many benefits of trauma-informed teaching. 'More is not better, more is confusing'. 'Your voice is a thread to safety'. 'Teach to Empower'. 'Trust the Yoga'. 'Show, Don't Tell'. 'Stay in Your Lane. 'Simple to understand. Simple to do'. 'Small choices. Small points of awareness. Small movements toward trauma recovery'. 'Be informed and be inspired'. 'Seeds planted'. 'It's body physiology'. Trust that you can build a sense of safety through your voice, your word choice, and your trauma-informed approach. Let's consider how.

## Building Safety

### Self-regulation

Your use of language can help someone become aware of their bodily sensations. Does noticing your leg muscles working or noticing you are holding your breath really matter? Yes. This ability to notice what is happening inside of you (interoception) is a first step to self-regulation. Being able to self-regulate can help someone feel safe in their body, which is a key step in trauma recovery (van der Kolk, 2015). Without knowing how you feel, it's a challenge to manage your responses. Someone can be stuck being reactive, unable to be proactive. That's a lot to put on using language. But fortunately, we are verbal creatures and well up to the task. Let's look at some ideas.

### Pacing

The pace at which someone speaks is affected by different factors. Where you are from (culture and geography), how comfortable you are with teaching various groups and with teaching yoga, your thoughts about leaving periods of quiet, and personality each can affect how quickly you speak. Why is pacing in a section on language? An image comes to mind of driving a car. You can drive too fast, too slowly, or just right for the conditions. The car doesn't change. The same words can be said at different speeds for completely different effects. Allowing someone time to process what you say, allowing time to explore the breath and movement, and allowing time to notice how it *feels* all contribute to how you empower someone to self-regulate. But wait. What about speaking too slowly for the conditions? The answer to that important question is: 'Your voice is a thread to safety'.

## 'Your Voice Is a Thread to Safety'

Stephen Porges' polyvagal theory lends strong science to what we already know from experience. One way mammals gauge safety is by listening to voices. Think growls. Think purrs. The takeaway point for safety is that from the prosody (tone and cadence) of your voice, most people can tell how you are feeling. Think of your voice as a thread to be followed back from wherever minds may have wandered. Or, perhaps more importantly, as a thread to keep someone's mind from wandering. Part of using your voice effectively is knowing how you sound to others and exploring your vocal options. The last section of Chapter 5 outlines some simple ways for you to fine-tune your vocal tool.

During the 'Final Stretch', a guided, body-based meditation, I am always talking (p. 167). Some have told me they don't listen but know I am there. Others listen, then don't, then come back. I thought, "Yes, indeed, a thread to safety." Talking about how fun the new aerial yoga studio is or how you love doing tree pose by a mountain stream or sharing ideas on why yoga is so helpful to trauma recovery is distracting. Someone shared, "I like your class so much better than Michael's. He just talks all the time." I smiled, as I also talk all the time. But I talk about noticing how something feels, about finding a new way to stretch today, or about how longer breaths out can lower blood pressure. Once you commit to maintaining 'your voice as a thread to safety', it becomes more natural to keep your trauma-informed voice going. Many strategies are woven throughout these chapters.

## Grounding

You can use language to show someone how to ground, which means being aware of the present. Grounding can happen as someone notices breathing and bodily sensations. Or grounding can happen when someone notices or senses something outside of themselves, perhaps a chair, the floor, or even a tree. Grounding can help rebuild a sense of time. As Pierre Janet, MD, observed in the 1890s, "Trauma is a disease of not being in the present" (van der Kolk, 2015). Someone can be stuck in the past, unable to enjoy the present and therefore unable to imagine a better future.

This teaching intention calls for specificity. "Okay, you may want to ground yourself," can be unhelpful and even agitating as someone may not know what you mean or how to do it. "Get grounded," can become: "As YOU breathe in, press down on your toes. As YOU breathe out, release." Another way to guide is to repeat a simple grounding phrase during a practice: "When you notice the muscles in your leg … when you notice the muscles in your leg, wiggle your fingers."

## Boundaries

Language can define time boundaries within which someone can explore bodily sensations and various simple breathing patterns. For example, "The suggestion is to practice three breaths here," defines a time during which someone can become curious. "Do I want to stay here for three breaths? Maybe I want to try today, or maybe I will try it next time. She said I am never stuck." Your simple words can create clear boundaries that build a sense of safety and in which to raise a stress threshold or widen a window of tolerance.

## Word Choice

Does it matter if you say shoulder problems or shoulder considerations? Does it matter if you call a breath 'the noticing breath' or 'the discomfort breath'? Daniel Kahneman, PhD, was awarded a 2002 Nobel Prize in Economics for research he did with Amos Tversky, PhD, showing how word choice framing a question affected decision making (Kahneman, 2013). So, yes it matters if you say shoulder problems or considerations. One way word choice can affect someone's sense of safety is words can be trauma triggers. A trauma trigger is a physiological response sometimes encoded as memory sensations and stored in the instinctive or emotional (subcortical) parts of the brain. Trauma triggers don't need words or thoughts, but certainly some words trigger a physiological response. Someone may not be consciously aware of their triggers. You may have thought, "Aha, feelings of guilt or shame can have unconscious triggers." Consider these potentially triggering words or phrases.

**The Body:** 'Squeeze your thighs' and 'blossom your buttocks' are yoga cues. There has to be a work-around to these phrases. Pat Ogden, PhD, offers that even the word *body* can be a trigger. Consider that "Notice where you feel the stretch in your body" can become: "Notice where you feel the stretch." Therapists told me that for some with eating or body image disorders, the word *weight* can be a trigger. "Shift your weight forward," can become: "Shift forward." As simple as that.

**Just Relax:** Relax is a word to consider expunging from your trauma-informed speech. At the time of trauma or abuse, some are told, "Just relax, you will like this." Relax can be heard as more of a command. Trust someone can experience a relaxed *feeling* through your trauma-informed teaching.

## Supporting Empowerment

The root word of empowerment is power. To experience trauma can be to feel a lack of power. So, part of trauma recovery and of building resiliency skills is regaining or strengthening feelings of agency. Teaching in a trauma-informed way means embracing the idea you are a guide, not the director of operations. There are clear ways your language can support feelings of both physical and emotional empowerment. Let's consider ways in which language can be directive, or how, should someone choose, a cue can be reworked to be empowering.

### Who's in Charge?

**Phrases to Take Anywhere:** David Emerson offers some simple and effective invitational phrases in his book *Overcoming Trauma Through Yoga* (Emerson, 2011). "When you are ready…" and "If you like …" are phrases that go with anything. Both phrases empower someone to make a simple decision. "Do I want to do as suggested? Am I ready to start now or would I like to wait?" Many studies continue to show that for behavior to change, someone needs to choose to do something (Stanley, 2019).

**It's a Hamstring Thing:** "You will feel this in your hamstrings." Well, you do not know where someone will feel a stretch. If your intention is to build body awareness and even some sense of curiosity, as Bessel van der Kolk, MD, says is key in trauma recovery, consider rephrasing. "You will feel this in your hamstrings," can become: "Notice where you feel the stretch."

**Close Your Eyes …** It's a common yoga cue. Yet closed eyes may make someone feel unsafe. They may think the pose or breath won't work if they don't close their eyes, or that this eye thing proves yoga isn't for them anyway. "Close your eyes," can become: "Eyes open or eyes closed, your choice. I keep my eyes open so I can see the door." But wait, not so fast. I said it that way for years to clarify that my reason was not to watch people. Then in a workshop someone shared that my saying I was watching the door only made her anxious. She said she kept thinking, "Why is she watching the door, what is she expecting might happen?" Hopefully, we are always open to refining our craft. So, I added, "Eyes open, eyes closed, your choice. I keep my eyes open so I can let you know if someone joins us." Then people started to comment how safe and welcoming that *felt*. Some people will open their eyes to check that you are doing as you had said.

**Don't Hold Your Breath:** It occurred to me one day as I said, "Remember to breathe," that I was missing the mark as I mindlessly repeated the directive I had heard for years. Again, I thought about a key point Bessel van der Kolk has shared in his workshops and writings: trauma recovery is about noticing something and developing a sense of curiosity. "Remember to breathe," became: "When you notice you are breathing … when you notice you are breathing, wiggle your fingers." You may notice that I pause to repeat the phrase, allowing someone the time to notice the *feeling*. I knew I was onto something when people wiggled their fingers, without my cueing it, on the other side of the pose. I remember I had wanted to say, "Yah, it works!" But I didn't.

**Do This, Not That:** "Keep a slight bend in your knees," tells someone what to do. It may seem an inconsequential point, as in "What's the big deal?" Well, if you are building a trauma-informed program, the more consistent and predictable you are, the stronger your program can be. Being nondirective applies to all things. "Keep a slight bend in your knees," can become: "Notice if you have a slight bend in your knees."

**Trust Me:** "This will make you feel better." Perhaps embrace the fact that you cannot know with certainty what will make someone feel better. In addition to possibly being a trigger, you may be setting someone up for failure. What if it doesn't make them feel better? Yet another thing they can't do. "This will make you feel better," can become: "Always breathe (or move) in a way that is comfortable to you today."

**Be Still:** "Find a moment of stillness." While I grasp the intention of this common yoga cue, it is not trauma-informed. For one, it lacks specificity, which can be distracting to someone not fully using the language part of their brain. For some, being still does not engender a feeling of safety, but rather stillness evokes a feeling of being trapped. You can't know, and sometimes they don't know. They simply feel that trauma imprint (no words) stored in the emotional or survival part of their brain (van der Kolk, 2015). "Find a moment of stillness," can become: "Find a way to stand as still as you would like to be today." People have told me they like that cue, as it made them think about how still they wanted to be. Then they could try to be that still. With your awareness and a little reworking of most phrases, you can build a sense of safety, support empowerment, and maintain simplicity.

**And, What's a Rule without an Exception?** Picture a room with a circle of yoga mats. Everyone has chosen to lie down at the end. "When you are ready, gently bend your knees and roll onto your side. Give yourself a few moments here." So far it sounds trauma-informed. Again, not so fast. Are you picturing people on their sides facing someone they may not even know? So, a clear directive can avoid this unfortunate face-to-face ending. "When you are ready, gently bend your knees and roll onto your right side, in the interest of personal space so you are facing away from each other." You have used your words to explain, in a simple and respectful way, why you are directing everyone to roll onto the right side. You may have noticed that this cue also shows you are managing the space for everyone's sense of safety. It's the little things, which turn out to be not so little.

## Choosing Words

A connotation is the extra meaning a word carries. Nuanced meanings are more subtle. Let's consider how to use these ideas to your trauma-informed teaching advantage.

**Lookin' Good!** If a trauma-informed intention is to build body awareness, then a trauma-informed pose is more about how it *feels* than how it looks to others. "That's really good, Kaya!" seems like an innocuous comment. But what does it tell Kaya and others? It says you are watching them. "Good job!" says you are judging them. Someone may think or *feel*, "Aren't I doing a good job? How come they didn't say that to me." But some people want and need attention, you may be thinking. Someone may need to be seen and to feel acknowledged, as they have spent a long time feeling invisible. Bessel van der Kolk, MD. and Gabor Maté, MD, note that trauma is when we are not seen and not heard (van der Kolk, 2015; Maté, 2022). You might consider making your comments observational, rather than value-laden. "Good job!" can become: "Kaya, it seems your tree pose feels strong today."

**Take Control:** I had always said, "You can control how you feel by controlling how you breathe." It sounded strong to me. But several wonderful yoga teachers strongly objected. By listening to my good counsel, I grasped the negative connotations of the word. "He was a controlling person," or "She thought she could control my life," or "The situation was out of control." Control connotes domination. The word managing has more of a work with me feel to it. "You can manage how you are feeling by managing how you breathe." Something to ponder as you choose your words. It's also another wonderful lesson in the benefit of being open to learning new things.

**Like a Pair of Old Slippers:** One day I used the word comfortable. It sounded right to me, so I kept using it. What is the difference between: "Move in a way that feels *good* today," and "Move in a way that feels *comfortable* to you today?" Well, what comes to mind when you hear the word comfortable? Perhaps a comfortable chair, comfortable seat, or comfortable shoes. You may 'plant a seed', the idea that doing simple breathwork or stretching can in fact be comfortable. Many continue to comment on how nice that word sounds to them, and some share they repeat it to themselves later. Or they say: "You said always move in a way that is comfortable to me today. So that's why I did it that way." Of note was they felt they needed my permission. But permission seemed the starting point they needed. "Always breathe in a way that is comfortable to you today," offers a simple variation. I knew it was working when a regular to our class told me, "I told my doctor, 'Look, it's my body, I know what feels right'."

**Don't Make It an Issue:** If you like, slowly say these three sentences aloud and pause between each one. I have an issue. I have a challenge. I have a consideration. Did they evoke the same *feeling*? Having an issue typically is not good. Meeting a challenge takes physical and emotional energy. "If you have a shoulder consideration, you might want to move your arm in a different way today." Why does the phrase also get repeated back to me? You may have already thought of it. The root word is considerate, which interestingly comes from the Latin word *consider are*, meaning to look closely or to observe. To be considerate of your shoulder has a gentle connotation. It may also create body awareness, another grounding opportunity.

**The Word Game:** Being aware of your word choices can keep you mentally engaged, which means you won't sound bored. Consider if a word or phrase comes equipped with a negative connotation. Or is there a positive nuance? When you find a word you like, there are two reasons to use it consistently. One is that with familiarity comes ease of understanding. The second is someone may hear your voice later in their minds when they need gentle trauma-informed guidance. You will find words that resonate with your style. Consider these examples of words that may bring extra and unintended meanings to your teaching.

1) **Drop it:** Drop often has negative connotations. Perhaps a few come to mind as you are reading: drop the ball, drop out, drop the subject now, and even drop dead. "Drop the chin toward your chest," can become: "As YOU breathe in, chin lifts. As YOU breathe out, chin releases."

2) **Lean On Me:** I had a wonderful yoga teacher who once suggested we try two things. If you like, put your hands on your hips. Feel your breath in, and as you breathe out, lean to one side. Now, as you feel your next breath in, press down on your hands, and as you breathe out, keep pressing your hands on your hips. Notice any difference? Leaning can feel like a collapse, while pressing creates some lift. Note to self: there are many words from which to choose.

3) **I invite you to ...** This phrase is common in yoga classes. It always made me prickle, and I finally figured out why. I understand the intention is to not be directive. But it always made me think, "Why do I need your invitation to practice a certain way?" The connotation is that without an invitation, you cannot attend. So, the phrase is not empowering. From other comments, I am not alone in finding this phrase unhelpful. This book has many ideas to consider for teaching with empowering or invitational language. None includes the phrase, "I invite you to ..."

**Practice Makes Perfect:** Oh, wait, we aren't trying for perfection. This idea struck me as quite important in cueing simple breathwork. "Take 3 breaths," can sound directive and harsh. I tried, "The suggestion is to practice 3 breaths." Using the word *practice* makes the breathwork sound judgement free and as though anyone can succeed. In cueing a movement, using the word practice brings the same message of support: we are all practicing. "Let's *do* 3 shoulder rolls back," can become, "The suggestion is to *practice* 3 shoulders roll back."

**Don't be Needy:** Here is another chance to use your words, literally, as you read these cues aloud. "If you wobble, just put your hand on the chair." Then say, "As you move to 'find your balance', you are building core muscles. Or today you may want to focus on the stretch and put your hand on the chair." Both cues are reasons to put your hand on a chair. But the first identifies weakness (wobbling), while the second supports a constructive choice (focusing on the stretch). If you are still playing, say this cue aloud: "If you can't reach your shoulder blade, then just put your hand wherever you can." Now say, "Find a comfortable place to put your hand. Different days, different stretches." Short, simple words can sneak into a cue: examples include can't, just, and need to. Short, simple words can work against empowering people.

**It's a Gift:** David Emerson's phrase "to give yourself a moment" beautifully captures how Dave teaches. Everything is crafted to support someone moving forward in healing. To me, that phrase is a gift of empowerment. You can give yourself the time you need. One day a regular came into class after her tough therapy session and said in a loud voice to me and anyone within earshot, "Okay, I need to give myself a moment … just to be." 'Seeds planted'.

## Knowledge Is Power

It took me a while to refine both why and how I wanted to provide information. Teaching simple breathwork provided my moment of insight. As noted, yet again, someone recovering from trauma may not be fully using the verbal parts of their brain or may be fatigued from sleep or pain challenges. Consider these ways to use your words. These strategies have worked in my diverse groups.

**Timing Is Everything:** Dumping extra words and ideas for the brain to process is not a strong start to a trauma-informed practice. But first guiding simple breathwork and movement to support resetting the nervous system is. Then later, a few times during or at the end of the practice when someone may be calmer and more open to learning, you can offer bite-size pieces of information. 'It's body physiology'.

**The Power of Choice:** Information offered with the intention of providing a choice can be empowering. "Long, slow breaths out *can* lower heart rate, lower blood pressure, and lower muscle tension. The suggestion is to practice 5 breaths." Where is the choice? I offered information without being directive. A slight change in wording keeps it fresh "The suggestion is to practice 5 breaths. Today, you may want to practice longer breaths in, which *can* be energizing. It's body physiology." Again, a single point of information creates a simple choice. 'Teach to Empower'.

**Point Positive:** As I was teaching older and injured veterans, the incarcerated, and refugees who spoke English, it occurred to me that they might like to know something positive they were doing for themselves. "You will feel this stretch in your upper back" can become: "Moving in this way can stretch muscles in the upper back." Consider two more simple points of information. "Warrior two is a power pose, strengthening your core and leg muscles," and "A longer breath in *can* be energizing."

## Maintaining Simplicity

### Teach Simply

If we heed the advice of B.S.K. Iyengar who devoted his long life to teaching and healing, then yoga as a felt experience should inform all we do. He advised in *Light on Yoga* that yoga cannot be explained in words, it needs to be experienced. And, as importantly, I would add that yoga as a felt experience should inform all we say. If this idea is new to you, perhaps give yourself a moment to consider that rather than talk about yoga, practice yoga. Iyengar's sage words inspired two phrases that I use in my trainings. 'Trust the Yoga' and 'Show, Don't Tell'.

**'Trust the Yoga':** 'Trust the Yoga' means you do not have to explain everything. Give someone the space, meaning the time and the mental space, to experience the yoga in their own way. Telling someone what they should feel or micromanaging how they move or breathe is not trusting the yoga. Sharing all you know probably will not improve their experience: 'More is not better, more is confusing'. I offer some comments I have received after my trainings.

- **From a yoga teacher:** "I live by 'Trust the Yoga.' In fact, I was feeling totally insecure about teaching a remote yoga class to my husband's coworkers. He just looked at me and said, "'Trust the Yoga' – isn't that what you always say? That yoga works?" Yes, that's what I say. And it worked! ~ N.K.
- **From a teacher working with a therapist:** "I cannot believe how at peace I am when I've let myself 'Trust the Yoga' when working with people in such pained circumstances. This woman just had her third miscarriage." ~ A.J.
- **From a therapist working with postpartum depression:** "Had my most agitated first day with a mom. I scrapped harder moves for more breaths and hand movements. While I was talking through a few rounds she shouted, "This feels AMAZING." ~ G.B.

'Trust the Yoga' has meaning beyond trusting you do not have to explain everything. The act of teaching also affects you. Look for more on 'Trust the Yoga' in the personal challenges section in Chapter 5.

**'Show, Don't Tell':** Having confidence in 'Trust the Yoga' sets you up to 'Show, Don't Tell'. Telling uses words to direct and to explain what will happen. For example: "You need to take long breaths out so you feel less anxious." Showing someone means using words to guide specific breathwork and body movements that, based on body physiology, can change a feeling state. "As YOU breathe in, fingers press ... As you breathe out, release the press." Or "When you notice you are breathing ... when you notice you are breathing, press down on your toes."

Okay, so 'Show, Don't Tell' greatly simplifies what you say, but it also can greatly complicate your day. Trying to teach simply is a challenge, as it goes against our often stream-of-consciousness, teacher/clinician-share-all approach. As Leonardo da Vinci is credited with saying, "Simplicity is the ultimate sophistication."

The phrases in Tables 11.1, 11.2, and 11.3 are based on these two key trauma-informed ideas: 'Trust the Yoga' and 'Show, Don't Tell' (p. 187).

**Expense Account:** Perhaps think of new words as being expensive. One way to conserve is deletion. Each time I taught a workshop, I would revise the scripts. I tend to be wordy. "As YOU breathe in lift your hands about six inches ... as YOU breathe out, bring your palms down to your legs," became: "As you breathe in, hands lift. As you breathe out, release." Extra words can divert attention from finding one's personal rhythm of breath and movement.

**How to Offer a Suggestion:** "I simply am offering suggestions," sets a nondirective tone. But folding the word *suggestion* into the cue simplifies it. "The suggestion is to step to the back of your mat." Or, "The suggestion is to take your hand off the chair as you 'find your balance'." Why not *my* suggestion? Again, *the* instead of *my* seems less directive. You can choose words to fit your style and personality. The important point, I suggest, is giving it some thought.

**Preamble or Pre-ramble?** These important ideas will be revisited in other sections, but you heard it heard it here first.

- **Oversharing:** There is no need to begin by listing your credentials. It may make you feel better, but it is extra words to process. As you teach in a trauma-informed way, someone should experience that you are qualified to teach.
- **Let Me Explain:** It is common for teachers, whether full-time yoga instructors or someone volunteering to share what they love, to begin a class with a lot of words. They can use words to justify why they are teaching, words to explain what yoga will do, words to share their mood today, and words to explain how someone might feel during the practice. Consider what you might feel if a teacher said (and one did), "Sometimes yoga can bring up a lot of feelings. If you get triggered, you can let me

know or you may want to leave the class." Someone may feel that they don't want a lot of feelings to come up, it sounds rather out of control. The teacher introduced to everyone that this class might be so upsetting someone may need to leave.

- **Sit Still and Listen:** Now consider the teacher starts class with a lot of words about a lot of things. *Feelings* of unease or disconnection can grow as nothing has been offered to connect someone to their practice. This idea of avoiding the pre-ramble also applies to ordering your cues. It is helpful to begin with an action (something to do), then a point of information, followed by another action. For example: "When you are ready, gently press one shoulder back … Then press the other shoulder back. A longer breath in *can* be energizing. As YOU breathe in …" This pattern is in the practice sequences.
- **Just Perk Up!** "You seem low energy. From how you are sitting, you seem depressed. Let's use some breathing and stretching to perk up. I know this really helps me on those days when I just feel blah. Do this with me." Did you notice a lot of words and no activity? In addition, what works for you is not relevant. Simplify: "If you like, let's practice the 'Tip-to-Toe' stretch 3 times. Today you may like to stand. Longer breaths in *can* energize. As YOU breathe in, arms stretch overhead. As YOU breathe out, arms release". 'Show, Don't Tell'.
- **Hey, Just Loosen Up!** "I can see by how you are sitting that you feel tense. I know you have a lot going on, and we talked about how today's session might be intense. Let's do something that always works for me. You should do it too." That string of judgements and potential triggers can become a simple and relevant suggestion: "The suggestion is to practice 3 shoulder rolls. Longer breaths in *can* lower blood pressure. When you are ready, …". Perhaps you are thinking, "Ah, 'Show, Don't Tell'."

**Avoid a Verbal Chase:** Using a cue to bring attention to the breath is trauma-informed. Consider, "Notice what it feels like as you breathe in … notice what it feels like as you breathe out…" While the teaching intention rings true, you may have sent someone on a verbal chase to find the words to describe what the breath in and the breath out feel like. "Notice what it feels like …" can become: "Feel the breath in … Feel the breath out." The teacher who taught that first cue told me, "Yes, this makes sense. There is more awareness with 'feel the breath in' because it gives an immediate focus, the breath! Fewer words, so simple!" Another verbal chase can be found in the cue, "Notice where your mind wandered." If you want someone to notice their breath, use your words to guide *feeling* the breath and not words leading somewhere else.

**It's in the Laundry:** You may have a lot of helpful information to share. But if you present things in a laundry list, whether the many benefits of yoga or instructions on what to notice (your heart rate, the temperature in the room, if you are losing focus as you breathe, where your mind wanders), you are not giving the verbal part of the brain a rest. You are distracting from the felt experiences of doing the yoga. "Is your chest rising or falling? Is your breath deep or shallow? Are you breathing in through your mouth or your nose?" is a lot to process at once. Consider choosing one idea to share. 'Simple to understand. Simple to do'.

**All Your Hopes and Dreams:** Setting an intention to start a yoga practice is common. A teacher in my teaching certification told me she opened her class with: "What is your hope for the next 45 minutes? Perhaps you want to connect with a friend or child. Just spending some time together. Maybe you are here for relaxation. Perhaps you want to just try something new. Whatever you choose as your intention, I want you to consider how that might inform or influence today's practice. Now, let's bring our awareness back to our breath. At your pace, I invite you to take three expansive breaths."

The ideas outlined here are lovely, but I mentioned it was a lot to think about. Someone may get stuck on what an intention informing a practice means. Did you spot the directive language and the word *relaxation*? Did you notice how the word *just* minimizes both spending time with someone and trying something new? Some cues lack specificity. How do I bring awareness back to the breath? And what is an expansive breath? We will circle back to some simple ways to set intentions in Chapter 9. Then you can find what suits your personality and the needs of your group. 'More is not better, more is confusing'.

## Literal and Body-based

How can you help someone focus their attention on their breath and bodily sensations? Quite literally, give the language part of the brain a rest. Let's consider some ways to communicate simply.

**Just the Facts, Ma'am:** As an old-time television detective used to say, "Just the facts, ma'am." Literal language and body-based cues keep it simple. "Feel the tension in your shoulders melt away," can become: "Notice where you feel the stretch as you move." "Breathe into the space around your spine," can become: "Notice what moves as you breathe." Use your words, that is use your language tools, to 'Show, Don't Tell'. "Reconnect to what your body is asking

of you," can become: "Move in a way that feels comfortable to you today."
"Ground yourself to feel release from the stress of the day," can become: "As
YOU breathe in, press down on your toes. As YOU breathe out, release."
And to spend even more time on this important idea, "Wrap your leg muscles
around your bones," can become: "When you feel the muscles in your leg …
when you feel the muscles in your leg, wiggle your fingers." If you are a yoga
teacher or have been to a yoga class, perhaps think of a cue you have used or
heard. How might you make it literal and body-based? That is, how would you
make it 'Simple to understand. Simple to do'? Again, in no way is language
filled with soft imagery wrong. But it can be distracting and one more thing
for a tired brain to ponder.

**Oh, Wait … What?** I used to say, "If you like, practice longer breaths out and
see what you think." The first part of the cue is nondirective, so that's okay.
But if my intention were to bring awareness to bodily sensations, then asking
what someone *thought* headed me away from the body. "If you like, notice if
a long breath out feels comfortable to you today." Use your words to say what
you mean.

**A Word of Welcome:** Well, perhaps a few words of welcome. An example is
to begin a class or to welcome someone later with: "Welcome. The suggestion
is to breathe and move in ways that feel comfortable to you today." That one
statement has an elegant simplicity. You have let everyone know you have no
expectations for their practice today, you have offered a body-based cue, and
you haven't engaged in information overload.


## Repetition and Consistent Phrasing

Let's consider why word repetition and consistent phrasing strengthen trauma-
informed teaching.

**The Power of the Pause:** It can be helpful to repeat your body-based cue
after a two-second pause. Simple repetition gives someone's brain a rest, while
keeping 'your voice as a thread to safety'. "If you like, put one or both hands
over your heart … Put one or both hands over your heart." You are giving
someone a moment to decide what they want to do today as well as the time in
which to do it, without cluttering up the airwaves with extraneous words and
distracting choices. Is a few-second pause helpful? Artur Schnabel, the gifted
pianist, is credited with saying, "The notes I handle no better than many
pianists. But the pauses between the notes – ah, that is where the art resides!"
Give yourself a moment to consider what happens during those pauses.

**And One More Time:** Another tool for creating simplicity in language is to use phrases consistently, so someone can become familiar with them and perhaps might even hear your voice later in their minds. A teacher told me she had chosen a few phrases to use consistently and "It's cool to hear the refugees repeat it back to me." "Different days, different stretches," may be something someone hears later in their mind as a gentle reminder that today may be different than yesterday or tomorrow.

**Find the Beat:** In a training, a therapist was role playing a resistant client. Their partner read breaks from the practice scripts (Appendix A). She told us after the exercise she was trying *not* to pay attention so as to be that resistant client. "But I felt myself being drawn in by the rhythm of their words, how the phrases kept repeating." She was quite surprised she had failed as the resistant client. Again, your voice can be a powerful teaching tool.

**********

**To Recap:** Language choices are key to every aspect of the GreenTREE Yoga® Approach: building safety, supporting empowerment, and maintaining simplicity. 'Trust the Yoga' and 'Show, Don't Tell' can guide your choice of language in developing trauma-informed strategies to meet your personal and professional goals. You will find relevant examples of these important ideas throughout the book.

## References

Emerson, David. and Hopper, Elizabeth (2011). *Overcoming Trauma through Yoga*. Berkeley: North Atlantic Books, p. 121.

Franklin, R. W., ed. (1999). *The Poems of Emily Dickinson*. Cambridge, MA: Harvard University Press, pp. 340; 466.

Kahneman, Daniel. (2013). *Thinking Fast, Thinking Slow*. New York: Farrar, Straus, and Giroux.

Maté, Gabor. (2022). *The Myth of Normal: Trauma, Illness, and Healing in a Toxic Culture*. New York: Avery.

Stanley, Elizabeth. (2019). *Widen the Window*. New York: Avery.

Van der Kolk, Bessel. (2015). *The Body Keeps the Score*. New York: Penguin Publishing, p. 21.

# 3
# The Yoga Space

## The Room

Consider that you are planning a special gathering. You want to ensure your guests have a quality experience and create good memories. What does a caring host consider? Perhaps the plan includes which rooms to use and seating arrangements. What are you serving to eat? Is there a centerpiece? Do you have lighting options? Is there background music? Do you mention if it is casual or formal? What time should they arrive and when does it end? Do you have a plan if Uncle Matthew and your cousin Aram pick up their political discussion fiasco of last year? I think you can see where I am going with this laundry list. A successful gathering is more than issuing invitations. It can be helpful to cast yourself in the role of manager as you plan your gathering.

## Building Safety

You are creating a space for social interaction with opportunities for trauma recovery and for building resiliency skills. The good news is with awareness and intention, you do not need a perfect situation. That's right, you do not need a perfect space to create many positive outcomes. I taught a pilot program in a cold hallway after hours in a women's clinic. Yet it worked so well that we got the veteran program funded. In fact, having a space in which things are not optimal offers an opportunity to practice simple breathwork and movement wherever you are.

The primary consideration continues to be building a sense of safety. A veteran came to my class after military sexual trauma therapy. "Can I just take my mat in the corner and lie down? I just need a place to feel safe." She covered herself with a soft cotton blanket and did not move the entire class. I will note that I never use the word safe in my classes.

DOI: 10.4324/9781003308836-5

## Arranging Physical Space

The following techniques outline ways to build a sense of safety in most physical spaces.

**Grab a Mat:** Prior to teaching veterans, I had taught at a fitness center. People put their mats in rows. We do what we know (think parenting) until we have cause to rethink it. I quickly learned that veterans with clinical diagnoses of PTSD do not like having people behind them. How did I learn this? They said, "We don't like people behind us." How does a circle or semicircle of mats build a sense of safety? Everyone can be seen, no one is behind anyone, and opportunities for social engagement are increased. I now teach all classes in a circle or semicircle of mats and/or chairs, whatever the group (veterans, refugees, the incarcerated, students, agency/school staff).

**Where Is the Door?** But I still did not have it right. At first, I was in the circle facing the door. I observed that the spots facing the door were always taken first. The class was not about me, so I relocated my mat with my back to the door, the spot no one wanted.

**The Humble Chair Can Do All That?** Consider that a chair is not only something on which to sit. A chair can help widen someone's window of tolerance in many ways.

- **Defines space.** Without mats, a chair easily defines personal space. A circle of chairs should allow enough room for someone to stand behind or to the side. Putting a chair at the back of each mat also gives more physical definition to the space.
- **Signals comfort.** A chair often is associated with comfort, thereby helping to build a sense of safety. Someone may think or *feel*, "I know this, how hard could it be?" A yoga mat can cause stress to someone new to yoga.
- **Empowers through choice.** A chair provides a choice. "Anything we do standing, you can also do seated." "Today you may want to have your hand on the chair and focus on the stretch. Or today you may want to take your hand off the chair to build core muscles. Different days, different stretches." 'Small choices. Small points of awareness. Small movements toward trauma recovery'.
- **Allows room for personal growth.** The option of a chair allows someone to practice balance or to pursue a stretch in a way that might not otherwise feel comfortable or safe. Today someone may do a standing balance with their hand off the chair for two breaths, while last week they did not.

- **Provides a time reference.** Someone might think, "Today I used a chair to focus on the stretch. Maybe next time I can focus on my core. Different days, different stretches." Again, cueing an action with the word *today* can help someone *feel* they are not stuck in yesterday or disconnected from today.
- **Grounds through body awareness.** Physically touching a chair also gives a visceral sense of grounding, taking advantage of the many sensory receptors in the hands. Interestingly, the expression "flying by the seat of your pants" came from early pilots. Without advanced navigation systems, they needed to rely on their physical sensations to gauge the plane's position (Ogden, 2006).
- **Normalizes.** A chair offers a way to normalize variations in abilities, whether within the group or for someone on different days. A class regular announced my substitute had not put out chairs, and he really would have liked the option. The chairs were easily accessible in the prop closet. Again, if everyone begins with a chair and your cues support using it "to focus on the stretch today," you have normalized using a chair.
- **Provides a visual cue:** Using the familiar chair gives a visual cue that yoga can be done anywhere – even in a kitchen or office. Later, the chair may be a reminder to give yourself a few moments for a short yoga break.
- **Reaching out for support:** Asking for help can be a challenge in trauma recovery. A chair offers a chance to reach out for support, quite literally, and to feel the benefits. These benefits can include feeling physical strength and feeling safe enough to try something new.

**Is This a Setup?** I was always early to my veterans' classes to arrange the room. Then I noticed women started getting to class earlier and earlier. I finally asked why. "We like to help set up." Another day a woman came after her group therapy and said, "I need to feel my body. Right now, I can't feel anything. Let me help you set up. I need to move." Then I noticed after class some of the women would bustle around putting the mats and carefully folded blankets in the closet. I remember saying, "You don't have to do that," to which one of them quickly replied, "We like to, it's part of the ritual." It also seemed to build a sense of community. I noticed the refugees liked to help set the chairs in a circle and arrange the food. Bessel van der Kolk reminds us that in 1893, Pierre Janet, MD, wrote about the "pleasure of completed action" (van der Kolk, 2015). Pat Ogden incorporates this idea in her Sensorimotor Psychotherapy® program, reminding us of Pierre Janet's insight that there is much benefit to physically completing an action someone could not at the time of trauma (Ogden, 2006).

**A Close-Knit Group:** Some traumas involve personal space violations. A trauma-informed approach reflects this sensitivity. Yet, be aware that for some, moving too close to others may happen as their personal space lines have blurred. As the manager setting up the room, know that having someone too close can cause stress. Making sure the mats or chairs are as well-spaced as the room allows is good planning. One young veteran explained to someone he had brought to class as he adjusted his chair, "I need room so when we do tree pose I can stand on the side of the chair. I need room."

**Don't Rock the Boat:** Why do I set up extra spaces if I think someone may join after the class has begun? Making room can itself become a point of distraction or anxiety. "If someone else comes in now, will I need to move my things again? Will they be too close? If I come later, will I be the one causing a fuss?" A trauma-informed manager minimizes distractions, infringements, and concerns.

## Creating Boundaries

You have set up the room and invited people to join. As with most things, there are things you can control and things you cannot control. And as with most things, it is important to know the difference.

**To Manage or Not to Manage:** Some situations you can and should manage. A maintenance person wanting to check the vents. That's a no. An intern who was told to rearrange the supply closet. That's a no. The Veterans Administration police who want to come in and talk with a woman about her service dog. That's a no.

What can you do about things you cannot control? Reframe them as opportunities to normalize situations, creating some wonderful 'Show, Don't Tell' teaching moments. One room in which I taught veterans created continuing opportunities. Initially, I would open our door and explain to the noisy custodians we were having a yoga class. Not only had I interrupted my teaching flow, but my annoyance detracted from the sense of safety. In addition, it was a lost opportunity to help someone raise their stress threshold.

**This May Happen …** So, what could I have done? A teacher working with Florida veterans taught me a simple approach. Identifying the possible interruptions or distractions at the beginning of class normalizes them and creates a boundary. A sudden clanging in a heating vent or bursts of noise from across the hall will not be complete surprises. What if I had said, all of which were true, "Oh, I know it's so hard to do yoga with that noise. But there is no other place we can go, believe me I have asked, so we are stuck here. And yes, I know the carpet is gross too." Instead, I chose to say, "Today there is a program across the hall, but we can still do our breathing and stretching, so it's not a problem."

The room in which I taught a women's class had construction happening literally outside the large windows. For over two years there were construction noises and workmen doing what workmen do. At the start of one class, I mentioned the men were working today. When there was a loud noise, I immediately looked at the woman new to class. She had frozen. What was remarkable to me was that she was looking right at me. Then she nodded and smiled, as if to say, "Oh, yes, you said this might happen, I'm okay." And on we went.

**The Abyss of the Unknown:** What if you do not know what might happen? It's covered with: "I am not familiar with this room. There may be some noises we don't expect from vents or sirens or people outside. But that's fine, we can still do our breathing and stretching today." You have set a boundary for knowing unexpected noises may happen. Others may be familiar with the space and offer ideas on what to expect. Another way to build community.

**Dual Processing Opportunity:** Pat Ogden uses the term dual processing to describe how someone can start to become triggered but can learn a new, less reactive response (Ogden, 2006). This dual processing can be done within the safe boundaries of your room. My biggest test, I mean opportunity, was when a new floor was installed in our room. Because of the outgassing of fumes, for four weeks of six classes a week I would repeat, "We can still do breathing and stretching, even with the door open and the fans on." After a few weeks of the open door, a highly anxious, older veteran wrote in the post-class evaluation comments: "I realize that I can now be okay with loud noises outside the door. It used to really upset me, but I am okay with it now."

## Props

**We Want Some!** One approach is people should feel they are enough and do not need props. That is not my approach. I feel trauma-informed props can be empowering and create opportunities for personal growth. The many values of the humble chair were outlined. One day women asked about the props in the closet. They were eager to choose blankets and bolsters. The men's class followed. They were curious. I heard a chorus of, "We want some!" So, they too chose blankets and bolsters to use. Arranging a bolster, a blanket, and perhaps a rolled-up mat became a key ritual to setting up personal space. To avoid the stress of too many things, I only use a few props. Blankets and bolsters, both with welcoming sensations of touch, continue to be appreciated. All soft, all optional. 'Small choices. Small points of awareness. Small movements toward trauma recovery'.

**When Is a Yoga Strap Not a Yoga Strap?** A six-foot strap with a buckle is a common yoga prop, wrapping and buckling being used to deepen a stretch around hips, arms, or legs. Feeling strapped in and unable to quickly navigate to another position can be triggering. I was in an office when someone said, "Oh, you're the yoga teacher. Your box of straps came in yesterday." I explained I didn't use straps in my classes. To underscore my point, I added I wouldn't even know what to do with them. A veteran said, "Yah, well my father sure knew what to do with a strap." I thought, "And there you have it."

**Empowered by Choice:** After the veterans demonstrated how much choosing props meant, I gave it more thought. The physical action of choosing props and then choosing how to use them can be grounding as it provides more sensory input. It also reinforces the physical feeling that this is now. "Last week, I did not use a blanket. Maybe today (or next week) I will try something different." Actively choosing also can build a sense of curiosity.

**Too Much of a Good Thing?** I was excited to continue exploring what props could bring to our program. I quickly found the limit. I had a bin of colorful mats, so I offered a choice of mats. That was, as they say, an epic fail. It was too many choices without the structure and familiarity of the mats already in a circle. Mat choices, take two. I put the mat bin by the door. The option was to choose a mat (various colors and thicknesses) to put over a mat I had already set out in our circle. I noticed no one did, so I stopped offering. Lesson learned, again and again: 'More is not better, more is confusing'.

**Opt-in/out Cards:** Some teachers put opt-in/opt-out cards for adjustments or oils at the front of everyone's mats. Cards are well-intentioned and not wrong, but cards are not trauma-informed. One reason is you aren't walking around the room making adjustments (pp. 84, 140–142). You also would be asking someone to draw attention to themselves, which can cause anxiety. The one time I do walk around a room is before our 'Final Stretch'. "I am going to walk around the inside of our circle now. You might like an ocean rock or a sprig of today's herb, fennel, in your palm. Feel free to take one of each." It isn't intrusive and I have identified the herb. It also doesn't cause someone the stress of having a card for all to see that says they don't want the nice thing you are offering.

## Five Senses: 'Be Informed and Be Inspired'

A veteran wrote this response after a practice: "I enjoyed the calm, quiet and harmonious atmosphere, the flowers, good smells from bread, and textures." The five senses are how we receive information from the world: sight, hearing, smell, touch, and taste. To review, we receive sensory signals, which are sent to various parts of the brain for processing. Then a motor response is sent back. Does the new information (stimuli) add to our sense of safety, or does it provoke a stress reaction? And do outside stimuli trigger internal stressors? Chapter 1 has more science on how we get information from ourselves and our world, and how trauma can disrupt signal processing.

Why should you care about the neuroscience of sensory stimulation? Well, as someone sharing the body-based modality of yoga, you have five sensory inputs to use or misuse. You can build a sense of safety and empower someone to self-regulate, or you can, unintentionally, introduce triggers into the space. Here is a good place to note you are not in a teaching bubble free of sensory stimulation. At some point, someone may have a negative response to what you say or do. But if you are using trauma-informed protocols that minimize potential triggers and empower someone to move through stressful feelings, it becomes an opportunity. Within that safe place, someone can widen their window of tolerance or raise their stress threshold. Ideas on how to manage stressful responses are in Chapter 4. The suggestion is to be informed. So, let's spend some time considering the senses.

### Sight

**The Eyes Have It:** Sight can be an important input to gauge safety. Consider that such prey animals as deer and rabbits have eyes on the sides of their heads to afford a wider field of vision to see danger. Those who have experienced trauma may suffer from hypervigilance or always being on guard for danger. As predators, humans do not have eyes on the sides of our heads. So being able to turn our heads quickly can be key in our sense of safety. A trauma-informed room setup reflects this awareness.

Another visual cue is lighting. Science has shown that flickering fluorescent overhead lights can be stressful, which is why many businesses and new school buildings install other forms of lighting. In one room, I kept the overhead lights off and brought in my own floor lamps, which one younger male veteran always arranged before class. It is important to keep the lighting constant. Sudden bright lights can trigger a release of adrenaline. If the room has windows to the outside and you know it is going to be getting dark, turn the lights on at the beginning of class so the light change is gradual. Of course, I learned this light lesson when I failed to plan. Also, the suggestion is not to turn off the lights for the last ten minutes of the class. Continually manage for consistency and predictability.

If you have the option, choose mellow colors for mats, blankets, and bolsters. One mat donation was bright pink with red lip designs. Interestingly, there is science behind color therapy. Do you have a favorite color, one that makes you feel calm or energized? Research shows that our bodies respond to colors because some of our cells have light-sensitive chemical switches. Some colors can cause certain enzymes to work more effectively, while others can affect what chemicals are produced (Doidge, 2015). I took several of the dissonant colors and patterns out of the mat line-up.

**Center with a Centerpiece:** Since I arrange my classes in a circle or semi-circle, I put a seasonal something in the center. Noticing a physical object can be grounding as it happens in the present. I may bring fresh seasonal flowers (nothing scented, for example, lilacs), dried grasses, small pieces of evergreens, collections of pinecones, shells, and special rocks from my travels. Someone might bring something and quietly add it to our centerpiece.

**Normalize:** There probably will be things in the space that you cannot control. "As you can see, this room is also used to store equipment for aerobics and weight classes. But we have enough room to do our practice." You have minimized the visual distractions by acknowledging the situation.

**It's a Two-way Street:** In one room in which I taught, there was a full window next to the door. Passers-by would stop and peer in at our all-women classes. Without comment, I covered the window, and the women thanked me. 'Show, Don't Tell'.

## Hearing

**Clangs, Bangs, Thumps, and Beeps:** To make more informed decisions about the effects of sound, a bit of science can be helpful. We know there are many types of sounds. Some sounds soothe, while others agitate. Such sounds as sirens, construction, or pounding bass music can disrupt your trauma-informed class. Soothing music and voices can activate muscles in the middle ear and also the social engagement system. Chapter 1 has more on this important idea. Interestingly, some types of traumas (and autism) decrease the functioning of the middle ear muscles. Someone may only hear the low tones, feeling overwhelmed with threatening sounds. And of course, some sounds are just annoying: bracelets jangling, a phone beeping text messages, or nearby conversations.

**It's Your Party:** If your trauma-informed intention is to build a sense of safety and to empower someone to self-regulate, then remember, it is your party. If you choose to introduce sounds into your room, do it with clear understanding. Again, 'More is not better, more is confusing'. Some considerations:

- **Low tones** can signal danger. Movie soundtracks and certain movements in classical music utilize this science.
- **Music with words** can be triggering or distracting. Chanting in other languages can be perceived as cult-like. And any words give the verbal part of the brain one more thing to do. Someone shared that the songs played by a teacher brought her back to high school. Not a happy place from her strong reaction.
- **Background music** played to mask deeper noises outside the room can in fact cause more agitation for the nervous system.
- **Music can calm,** making someone more open to noticing bodily sensations and their breath.
- **Calming music** to one may be agitating to another. A regular class participant brought in music she said was a great fit for our class. I will skip to the end: a very poor idea to play something you have not heard. Women in my refugee classes wanted music and offered to bring some. I looked around at women from 15 different tribes and countries, and said, "Let's go with quiet and focus on our breathing."
- **Music can distract** from emotions, physical sensations, and breath awareness. Many teach without music, preferring the focus to be on what is being experienced. Fewer sensory distractions can mean more attention to the felt yoga experience.
- **A Real Yoga Class:** I prefer to teach without music. But veteran comments indicated they felt it was not real yoga without music. I gathered some data. I began to play soft music, gentle tones, no words, no banging, no drumming. I included a question on the optional after-class evaluations. Everyone liked the music, except someone who wrote, "I don't care." Given that was the least positive comment, I continued to play it. People asked me for the names of the CDs. An older veteran wrote in her comments, "I enjoyed the lovely Native American flutes as a background to Yael's gentle guidance." How does one decide? Well, my suggestion is to give it some thought. If you know your group, use that information. If

you do not know your group, consider your trauma-informed options and go from there.

**Let's Hear it for Grounding:** I learned that using metal chimes or metal singing bowls can cause some with tinnitus (ringing in the ears) extreme discomfort. Exposure to gunfire often creates hearing issues. I then learned that using glass bowls does not bother those with tinnitus. There can be fun ways to use several different sounds to ground through awareness. To avoid startling anyone, always say what sounds you will be introducing. "I will play three tones. If you like, notice if they are different." Or "I will play three tones. When you can no longer hear them, press down on your fingers." But again (and again), 'More is not better, more is confusing'.

**What Just Happened?** Playing music for only the last ten minutes may be distracting, as it is a new sensory input. The suggestion is to keep consistent lighting and sounds for the whole class. If you play music, keep it at the same volume (low) throughout the class. If you have problems with the music system, stop playing the music. Trying to fix it interrupts your teaching flow. And annoyance is not a good look on someone sharing yoga.

## Smell

**No Thought Required:** It's worth mentioning again that smell is the strongest encoder for memory. The olfactory neurons detect smells, and the signals are sent directly to the amygdala, and a response follows. The information is not first routed to the neocortex, or higher-level thinking. You smell something and can have an immediate, visceral response. The sense of smell is the only sense that works this way. Good information to have when bringing smells or scents (scented candles, incense, sage smudge sticks) into a room. Add that piece of science to the fact that someone may not even be consciously aware that a scent or smell is a trauma trigger. Again, the smell may be encoded as a nonverbal memory that elicits a physical response with no thought. A cinnamon smell may trigger the feeling or the bodily sensation of that traumatic holiday visit.

**But the Label Says ...** Based on science, it makes sense to limit the olfactory stimulation, which means not wearing perfumes, aftershave, or highly scented creams. Let's talk about smells that can fill a room. Incense by design wafts everywhere. Burning incense, sage sticks, or scented candles imposes your choice of smell on everyone. And someone may have respiratory considerations irritated by strong smells or smoke. A yoga teacher happily told me, "Oh,

I just light it before class and wave it all around so when people come in the rooms smells like sage." Hopefully, you can see how that approach is well-intentioned but does not meet the trauma-informed sniff test. Essential oils also quickly disperse throughout a room. Know that if you give one person a few drops, those around them will be experiencing the same oils. An exception comes from my experience at our state prison, which I share on page 69. Instead of highly aromatic incense or essential oils, perhaps offer sprigs of fresh herbs or evergreens.

Recently, someone reminded me of something I had done four years previously. The Warrior Renew group (Katz, 2014, and p. 173) had walked to the yoga room so everyone would know where to go the next week. I had left a welcoming note on the door with tied bunches of fresh lavender to share. The woman told me she had hung that lavender from her car mirror, for weeks feeling (and smelling) the warmth of my welcoming invitation.

**If You've Got It, Flaunt It:** There are many ways to use the five senses to ground, including the sense of smell. I know several therapists who keep rosemary plants in their offices, offering clients some to roll between their fingers. I used to offer fresh herbs just before our 'Final Stretch'. Some placed it on chests, in palms, or even under noses. Then it occurred to me that offering at the beginning of class could be a lovely way to help ground (sight, touch, smell). I noticed people put the herbs at the front of their mats and would sometimes pick them up during class. 'Show, Don't Tell'.

**Is Monday Wash Day?** Let's talk mats and blankets. New mats can outgas smells for a while, so you may want to air them before using. Over time, mats used by a group can get, well, smelly. Donated mats also can benefit from being included in wash day. Mats may do well in a washing machine (hot water, unscented detergent, and bleach) and then line dried. Of course, do your own test washes as mat materials vary. Blankets may need to be washed. Again, using unscented detergent or unscented fabric softener sheets can avoid smell triggers.

## Touch

**It's Texture Week:** Science and experience tell us that we have a high concentration of sense receptors in our hands, feet, and lips. With that fact in mind, I will offer something to hold in the palms for our 'Final Stretch'. It is interesting to vary it each week. "It's texture week," accompanies feathery fennel leaves. Or I may offer a smooth shell and a rough stone, without any prompts. Of course, I had a misstep, well-intended but not well-thought-out. Turns out that the pinecones I had collected from a local canyon upset someone with sensory processing considerations. It's a process. I now only use older cones with no sticky sap.

**No Really, How Does It Feel?** When choosing blankets, consider the feel of the material. I have seen blankets used as covers while lying down, as shoulder wraps while seated, or as rolls under the back or knees. Some cotton blankets can be soft and welcoming. The dark wool blankets I found in a supply closet reminded me of horse blankets. I purchased my own soft cotton blankets to share. If you have the luxury of choice, let the literal feel of something guide you. I felt good about my investment when a woman covered herself and said, "Oh, I just feel so snuggled in, I may stay here all afternoon."

**Step It Up:** Someone may choose to do yoga in bare feet, providing many opportunities for increasing sensory experiences to build body awareness and to ground in the present. Including mats with varied textures can add to your teaching opportunities. "If you like, stand with one foot half on and half off the mat." On a thicker mat, pressing down firmly on the toes has a different feel than on a thin mat. Ah, so many simple sensory experiences to be explored.

## Taste

**Let's Do Lunch:** Science and common sense tell us eating together can stimulate the social engagement system, therefore helping to build a sense of safety. I started baking for classes long before I had read Stephen Porges' inspiring work, as I think baking provides several positives. One, it shows a desire to create a connection with the group. I might share this recipe was my mother's, I picked these raspberries in my yard, or I flew home with these organic blueberries from my sister's fields in Maine. It also helps build a sense of curiosity. People would ask, "Oh, what did you bake us this week?" Again, taking the time to share food can help build a visceral feeling of safety. 'Show, Don't Tell'.

**It's All About You:** Obviously, how you share food is an opportunity to express your personality. For one-hour classes, I bring baked goods or perhaps squares of dark chocolate, with and without nuts, and seasonal fruits. I offer the food as people are filling out the optional after-class evaluations. I share foods with a theme to highlight seasonal changes: pumpkin bread, peach cake, raspberry muffins, apple cinnamon muffins, and carrot cake. With refugee and immigrant groups, we begin by sharing food during the ten minute

'Opening Connections' as I know some have not had time to eat or may not have extra food at home. With veterans, we end with food. Once a young veteran asked to start with some of whatever I had baked, stating that he really just came for the food. In some classes, I would add the option of a variety of hot teas to go with the baked treats after class.

**More Points of Connection:** In some classes, people brought teas and herbal coffees to share. Someone brought fresh honey to add to our tea bin. Veterans sometimes would bake for us and share recipes; refugee women would bring food to add to the counter of treats. In classes in which food was not an option, I really felt the lack. At the state prison, I had to settle for leaving the guys with an inspirational quote on a small piece of paper to take back to their cells.

**********

**To Recap:** Consider that you are planning a special dinner gathering. You want to ensure your guests have a quality experience and create some good memories. You consider what any good host does in planning a successful get together. With some thought, you can find ways to create a space that expresses who you are and meets the needs of your groups by building safety, supporting empowerment, and maintaining simplicity in all aspects of your program. Let 'Show, Don't Tell' be your guide.

## References

Doidge, Norman. (2015). *The Brain's Way of Healing.* New York: Viking Press, p. 121.

Eagleman, David. (2021). *Livewired: The Inside Story of the Ever-changing Brain.* New York: Vintage Press, p. 92.

Katz, Lori. (2014). *Warrior Renew: Healing from Military Sexual Trauma.* New York: Springer Publishing.

Ogden, Pat. (2006). *Trauma and the Body.* New York: W. W. Norton and Company, pp. 168; 205; 273.

Van der Kolk, Bessel A. (2015). *The Body Keeps the Score: Brain, Mind, and Body in the Healing of Trauma.* New York: Penguin Publishing, p. 218.

# 4
# Classroom Management

At first glance, a section on classroom management may seem odd. But given that building a sense of safety is the chief consideration in any trauma-informed setting, the human dynamic takes on added significance. In Chapter 1, we discussed the field of Interpersonal Neurobiology (IPNB), as well as the polyvagal theory, both of which explore how our personal interactions affect our biology. What does this research have to do with managing people? As it turns out, a lot. A trauma-informed approach goes beyond breathwork and yoga poses. As Bessel van der Kolk, MD, notes, "Social support is not the same as merely being in the presence of others. The critical issue is *reciprocity*: being truly heard and seen by other people around us, feeling that we are held in someone else's mind and heart" (van der Kolk, 2015). One veteran wrote in her after-class evaluation, "Yoga with Yael is like family." How did I manage that? I practiced the tried-and-true approach of 'Show, Don't Tell'.

If you want someone to not be disruptive, to feel safe, and to experience social connection, you need to be aware of the group dynamic. If you want someone to feel less resistant, less triggered, and less nervous, you need ways other than telling them. "You are safe," and "Yoga will make you feel better," and "You all need to be quiet during yoga," are examples of telling. Let's consider ways to 'Show, Don't Tell'.

## Building Safety

Where do you start? Chapter 3 discusses how to manage the physical space using building a sense of safety as a guide. As you might then expect, managing the people in that space is guided by the same trauma-informed principles. Any unease you may feel about exercising your managerial skills may have to do with personality, age, or culture. If you are younger, setting boundaries may

DOI: 10.4324/9781003308836-6

be a challenge. In some cultures, younger people are taught to respect their elders and teachers. Yet consider that you can manage in a style that is always respectful.

It may seem this management idea is yet another thing to consider in a growing list. And you would be correct. Yet consider that a single disruptive person can have a cascading effect and ruin the experience for others. One male veteran said to me, "That other teacher has no classroom control. You have great control." An interesting observation given that I am a small, soft-spoken woman, the other teacher a large male. Yet his perception was I had control. Why? Certainly not because I said I was in charge, but because I showed I could manage. I do have the advantage of having taught in classrooms from preschool through college (sciences), so classroom management is engrained in my approach.

Instead of thinking of classroom management as one more thing to consider, reframe it as one more trauma-informed tool. The following are some strategies I have used over many years and with many groups. You have your own personality, as do your groups. Adapting these techniques can be a solid place from which to build your own program. You are creating a place in which someone can have powerful and enlightening experiences. The alternative is that you fail to reframe yourself as a classroom manager and only react to situations as they unfold before you and everyone else.

## Predictability and Consistency

Hypervigilance, or being in a continual physiological state of arousal feeling danger always lurks, is not uncommon and fuels strong startle responses in someone in trauma recovery. You can help minimize arousal with predictable and consistent responses to such things as someone telling upsetting stories, making unsolicited requests, coming late or leaving early, interrupting with chatter or phones, or being triggered or resistant. If you have considered your responses as a part of your class plan, you become proactive and not reactive. Let us count the ways.

**Boundaries:** Clear and consistent boundaries help build a sense of safety. One boundary is on cell phones. "Please put your cell phones on silent, and no texting or calls while we practice. This time is for taking care of you." Before I clearly stated the boundary, people would take calls, stand outside the room talking loudly, then rap on the door to come back. Texts during our 'Final Stretch' would startle someone on the next mat.

**A Place to Call Home …** Someone having a favorite spot is not uncommon. But location takes on additional importance in a stressed group. As the manager, you can save someone's place. Would we do this in a typical yoga class? I have never encountered a teacher saving a place, but again, this class is not typical. Once a long-time participant entered the room, saw someone in his spot and simply left. I texted later to explain I would make sure the space was open next time. He did come back, as he trusted me to do as I had said. The place by the post had been saved by simply putting an extra chair on the mat. No words were exchanged. The message to others: you know and respect individual needs, and you set safe boundaries.

**My Back Is Killing Me:** Some teachers will ask, "What would you like to work on today?" This seemingly innocuous question can signal you have no plan, even if you do. Someone could think, "I didn't come for their knee issues, I came for me. Now what's going to happen?" It is more trauma-informed to avoid wide-open questions. Within a predictable class structure, you still want to be positive when someone asks, "Can we do low back today? My back is killing me." Your response: "Yes, of course. We will stretch areas around the back first. Always move in a way that is comfortable for you today." Then, as you do the predictable class sequence, you can mention how the stretching or strengthening helps the back. Someone with back considerations feels supported. Someone without back considerations feels informed. You also can add, "And, I will be happy to talk with anyone about more back stretches after class." Some ideas are on page 173.

**Aren't Yoga Classes Quiet?** I taught veterans with military sexual trauma for many years. A trauma-informed manager monitors the flow of interactions in the room. The flow can bring the healing effects of social connection, or it can bring distracting, triggering chatter. A comment showed me the need for a boundary. In the middle of class, women started talking. A regular participant visibly cringed. Then sounding agitated she said, "Look, can we just get back to the yoga?" I learned that I had not done a good job.

I had to think about how to handle this very chatty group, as I did not want to say, "Okay, no talking." Social connection also can be created as you breathe and move together. The next class I said, "Okay, if you like, today we are going to notice our long breaths out." And during the class I would cue, "If you like, notice your long breath out." I was truly amazed at the change. There was much less chatting and no conversational interruptions. With gentle reminders to notice long breaths out if you like, the change continued in the following weeks. Chapter 10 explains a different approach for refugee and immigrant groups.

**A Gentle Redirect:** Veterans with PTSD often would begin to share war stories, literally telling stories of war as we sat in our circle before class. Then, someone would try to top the previous story. One day I clapped my hands on my legs. "Hey, who has a dog story?" A couple of people rallied, and we had some smiles. But it was then necessary to set another parameter. "Who has a dog story in which the dog doesn't die?" Yes, I had to say that every week. But the redirect worked well. I was at the door when a veteran in our circle clapped his hands on his legs. He interrupted the start of a war tale with, "Okay, who has a dog story?" We looked at each other and smiled.

**A Clear Explanation:** Sometimes, you need to be more direct. "We are going to use this time to do some simple stretching and breathing. We can hold our stories until the end." You respectfully are showing you have created a consistent and predictable space. During a time of lively political feelings, I had to implement a blanket, "No Discussion of Politics" rule. I would laugh and simply say, "Oops, our yoga room is a politics-free zone. Taking care of my nervous system." It became a joke, and others would offer reminders as needed.

**My House, My Rules:** House rules can become an issue when a teacher is invited to a facility with its own rules. In a prison, house rules are the rules. But in other situations, there may be ways to establish that you are creating a space, literally, in which to practice yoga. In a school or clinical setting, a teacher, coach, or clinician may want to dictate the behavior during your yoga class. Prior to class, you can discuss which rules support your trauma-informed intentions and which rules do not. The takeaway point is that you have the right and, yes, the responsibility to find a respectful way to manage *your* class in a trauma-informed way.


## To Welcome

**Tell Us About You:** Some teachers will ask about concerns. Teachers have told me, "Oh, that's a really good point. I mean I knew that, and I don't know why I didn't think about it." That really good point is someone who has experienced trauma may not want to self-identify as having triggers or trauma concerns. They also want to please and not attract attention, often long-practiced strategies for avoiding stressful situations. Do you really want someone to have to say, "Don't touch me or I will freak out"? Again, someone may be unaware of their triggers or may believe they've gotten over them. The workaround is that instead of asking, either verbally or with a questionnaire, simply teach with trauma-informed protocols.

**Let Me Tell You About Me:** There is another reason not to ask about triggers or concerns. As I mentioned, some may share their trauma tales or tales of others to create a social connection. Yet, it is your space to manage and into which you have invited others. Again, it is your party.

## Interruptions

**All the Comings and Goings …** Someone may be arriving by car, mass transit, or walking from another place on site, as in treatment centers or prisons. Someone may have control over arrival times. Sometimes they do not. What you have complete control over is your response. For someone in the early stages of trauma recovery, it may take everything they have to get to your door. I was about to close the door to start class. A woman stood there, making no motion to enter. She stared at me with a flat affect. She then said in an equally flat tone, "Well, you called. I am here." Still, she was not moving. It seemed that it had taken all she had to get herself to the door.

When someone came late, I used to explain it was fine to come anytime and I was glad they could join us, which was itself an interruption. It took me a while, but I finally settled on one of two greetings, always said with a smile. "Welcome, come when you can, leave when you need to," was one. I noticed someone would quietly find an open spot, feeling no need to apologize for taking up space. The second greeting, "Welcome, find an open spot. Aways breathe and move in a comfortable way," also provided a gentle reminder to everyone.

But the "leave when you need to" needed some refinement. Do not expect people to understand either your intentions or the needs of others. I end longer classes with the 'Final Stretch' (p. 197). Envision a room of people, most with clinical diagnoses of PTDS, choosing to lie on mats with eyes closed, listening to me. Then, someone puts on shoes, rolls up a mat, walks to the closet, and looks for keys. Yes, completely disruptive. I added, "If you need to leave, now would be the time before we start our 'Final Stretch'." I also suggest they leave all their props in the spot, minimizing disruption. Well, problem not totally solved.

If someone does choose to leave after everyone is settled, a trauma-informed manager calls a play-by-play. "Okay, John is getting up to leave now, so you may hear him putting on his shoes. Just leave your mat if you like, John. Okay now I am opening the door and John is leaving. Now I am closing the door and going back to my mat." Sounds silly, actually quite silly, but it is not. It shows that you are monitoring the room. It explains the noises. Micromanaging? Perhaps, but it works to build a sense of safety. 'Your voice is a thread to safety'.

**Another Interruption:** Sometimes staff may attend, sitting in the back of the room chatting, unaware they are being rude. You have set out extra mats. A trauma-informed manager says, "You are welcome to join us, but if you need to chat, please go outside." Interns or volunteers may attend. It is appropriate to speak with them before or after class to encourage them to be on time. Someone arriving late is still an interruption. Manage what you can.

**The Art of the Reframe – From Interruption to Team Building:** Social connection is something to build at every opportunity. I found someone might text me if they were going to be late. "Looking for a parking spot." Or "I will be there in ten minutes." So right before I started class, I would check my phone and let everyone know that Angela was going to be joining us soon. Note I did not say late, I said joining us. A knock on the door was expected. I realized this sharing was building community: I am part of this group, I will let them know I am coming. Someone cares.

If someone texted they would be missing class, I would tell the group, "Neela won't be joining us today but says hello." I noticed more people started texting. I was able to give updates before the class, without sharing any personal information of course. Someone texted to say she did not want to interrupt as she was running late, so she would not come. I texted to please join when she could. I let the group know Rajaa would be joining us. When she arrived, she had a big handful of fresh mint. I invited her to walk around the inside of our circle to share it: not an interruption, but a lovely addition to our class. Predictable and consistent.

**Where was I?** You are in the middle of a five-part breath. Someone knocks on the door. My suggestion is to open the door immediately as knocking is a distraction. You open the door and say, "Welcome." The person goes to the open mat/chair you have included in your circle. Now you have a choice. You can be annoyed, creating stress in the room. Or you can say, "Okay, I am not sure where we were. Maybe some of you kept going while I got the door. ('Plant a seed'.) But let's do the five breaths from the top." You also have modeled moving with ease through disruption.

**A New York Minute:** We have different concepts of time, varying by culture and even parts of a country. You know your group. Sometimes at the end of class, I mention I hope everyone can join for the whole practice next time – the starting part, the middle, and the end. It's a gentle reminder there is a flow to the class. Some refugee trainings stress the new culture's sense of time. If a start time is noon, it means noon and not any time before one. Someone with PTSD or other unresolved trauma may be working to reactivate the time-sensing parts of their brain. Groups for which this reminder is not appropriate are those who do not control when they move. Some residential facilities have set class schedules, and prisons have prescribed times of movement.

**Be the One-Minute Manager:** A quick way to quiet a room is: "If you like, put one or both hands over your heart … Put one or both hands over your heart. The suggestion is to practice 3 breaths. Listen for your breath in … Listen for your breath out." (*Say 3 times slowly.*) Once someone put their hands over their heart and looked at me, as if to say, time for quiet. Another quick way to quiet a room is: "You may want to notice your long, slow breath out as we practice 3 breaths. As YOU breathe in, arms stretch up … As YOU breathe out, arms release." (*Say 3 times slowly.*) Pairing simple breathwork with movement replaces random chatter with a group feeling of synchronized breathing and movement. 'Show, Don't Tell'.

**Be Direct:** A direct boundary can be an effective boundary. "Let's use this time to do our yoga practice. We can chat after class." My favorite story of the direct approach is from my fourth class at our men's state prison. Picture about a dozen men in a semi-circle of mats around me. In the middle of the practice, two men, and I will note for the sake of the story, both large men in shorts and one with his shirt off as well, tattooed from head to toe, were talking and distracting me, and probably others. I turned and said, "Hey, do I need to separate you chatty boys?" I laughed. They laughed. The question was the teacher in me managing my space. In thinking about it later, I noted to myself that I would not have done that on the first day, not before I had experienced feeling very appreciated and welcome and safe in this group of guys.

**The Individualized Approach:** You have another option should someone become disruptive and unresponsive to your respectful efforts to redirect. Someone who had been coming to our class for a year burst into the room, talking and moving in a dysregulated manner. We invited her to join, but she was not able to hear us. I spoke softly as I guided her out, suggesting that another time she could practice with us.

## Managing Responses

Someone may feel anxious in a new situation or become triggered. Others may feel resistant to new things. Consider these easy ways to address such emotional responses without calling attention to someone.

## Anxious or Triggered Responses

A common question is what yoga tools are available if someone is triggered or becomes agitated during a class or a clinical session. Some clinicians use client body language to guide their sessions. A trauma-informed teacher and health care provider can do the same. Make your suggestions to the group, providing all with the opportunity to practice self-regulation skills. There are varying degrees of being triggered. Let's start small and work our way up.

**It Started as a Little Thing:** You notice signs of agitation. You can seamlessly weave these yoga breaks into your yoga class flow or clinical session.

- **Grounding or Five-part Breath with Finger Movements:** Short breath-work ideas to ground are in Chapter 7: At-the-Ready and the Five-part Breath sections. You may find a few favorites to have at the ready. The suggested breath fact for grounding is: "Long, slow breaths out *can* lower heart rate and lower blood pressure."
- **In a Heartbeat:** "If you like, put one or both hands over your heart … Put one or both hands over your heart. When you notice your heart beating, switch hands." The simple act of feeling your heart beating can be grounding and calming.

**Shake It Out:** If nervous energy or anxiety levels seem to be increasing, you can provide a (two-minute nervous system reset. Building on the idea of gently shaking the fingers on one hand, you can offer the 'Silly Shake and Stretch' (p. 220). I was inspired by the seminal work of Peter Levine, PhD. As his research tells us, shaking is one way mammals release stress (Levine, 2010). James Gordon, MD, founder of The Center for Mind/Body Medicine, uses movement in his programs to help populations with severe traumas (Gordon, 2019). The 'Silly Shake and Stretch' usually makes people smile, which can be a stress release. People seem reassured when I say, "Oh, laughing is good. Long breaths out *can* lower heart rate and lower blood pressure." 'Silly Shake and Stretch' may not be appropriate for mixed-gender groups.

**Don't Shake It Out:** Please note that for some, shaking a hand can be uncomfortable as it may signal an out-of-control feeling, or it may simply hurt. I expanded the cueing for a silly variation.

> If you like, gently move the fingers on one hand or shake that hand … Then gently move the fingers on the other hand or shake that hand. You may like to gently move or shake one foot … Then gently move or shake the other foot. Can you move or shake one hand and one foot? Notice is you smiled. Now if you like move or shake the other hand and the other foot.

The suggestion is to cue gently moving the fingers first, so someone starts with a feeling of safety and can easily stay there, as opposed to beginning with shaking and experiencing emotional or physical discomfort. Set up for success. Now you have a few moments of quiet after the laughing, shaking, and silly comments. 'In a Heartbeat' (p. 162) or 'Listen for Your Breath' (p. 78) can provide that reset.

**The Art of the Reframe:** Even if 'Final Stretch' (p. 167), the final guided body-based mediation, is done, your managerial tasks may not be.

- **Anyone Have a Tissue?** You notice someone is teary during 'Final Stretch'. Before you cue the ending, mention to the group: "Sometimes as we breathe and stretch and reduce muscle tension, things can come up. These feelings can mean you had a good practice. It may be helpful to talk with someone but know these feelings are not uncommon." Then continue and cue the usual ending. Usually, it is distracting to ramble on about the benefits of yoga. But normalizing emotions is an exception, and it may be helpful to others as well.

- **Not Quite What I Expected:** A woman sat up after 'Final Stretch'. "Wow, I couldn't feel my fingers until we just did that finger breath," she said watching her hand as she moved her fingers in 'Thumb to Fingertips Breathing' again (p. 134). Then she put away her props and stood there, not moving. She started to cry. It happens. Yoga supports reconnecting to physical sensations and emotions. What was numb becomes felt. Experiencing these new feelings can be upsetting. I said, "Would you breathe with me?" She nodded. I suggested she stand against a post. "If you like, press one shoulder back, then press the other shoulder back. Notice the back of your head resting on the post." I then cued all five breaths as we did them together. "You may like to practice long, slow breaths out. As YOU breathe in, arms lift … As YOU breathe out, arms release." I did not say anything. I waited. She simply nodded as if to herself and said, "Okay." She got out her keys and left. Sometimes you do not have the opportunity. A 36-year-old veteran was fully engaged during the practice. He texted me later saying, "I felt myself getting all teary, but I didn't want to cry." He didn't return.

- **Oh No, I Went to Sleep!** Someone may doze during 'Final Stretch', especially if sleep or pain challenges cause fatigue. My normalizing comment: "You seem to have had a good practice today." But if someone does not notice others moving around, avoid startling them. I will suggest a friend gently put a hand on their arm. Or I will. Strong startle responses are not uncommon, so be aware that sudden defensive movements might occur. But it can be more stressful to wake in an empty room. Before class, someone might announce to all that they are going to fall asleep today, like always. That's your cue to ask how they would like you to let them know class has ended. Take every opportunity to build safety and support empowerment.

- **I Don't Know What to Do:** I have had several people tell me the yoga practice made them so relaxed (not a word I ever use) that they felt upset. One young woman said, "I don't know what to do with that feeling. I don't like it." Again, I offer that doing yoga can reduce tension in the body and in the mind, which can mean you had a good practice. But it may be helpful to talk with someone about the feelings that may have come up. That's it. 'Stay in Your Lane'.

**A Bigger Issue:** Yoga is not an instant cure. While a simple five-part breath can lower heart rate and blood pressure in real-time, it may not be enough to override larger issues. Chapter 5 covers the importance of establishing a protocol and identifying your support system if someone needs to leave the room. Establishing that protocol before you teach is part of a strong management plan.

## Resistant Responses

**I Don't Want To ...** Someone may say, "I can't do this today," or "I don't even want to be here." As with all trauma-informed situations, your response should be predictable and consistent. You offer sitting on a mat or chair. "If you like, you can do the parts of the practice that feel comfortable to you today." One day a veteran burst into the room before class, almost dragging another woman. "Tell her. Tell her it's okay to just come to our class and just sit there. Tell her that's okay." It was interesting that I did not need to tell her, others chimed in. In all my years of teaching, giving someone control over how they practice has only failed once. Someone was made to attend my class before she could get more pain meds. I know this because she stomped into the room and told us, then sat and glared at me. When the distracting comments started, I suggested she could leave and rejoin us another day when she thought it would be a better fit.

If you are calling to invite someone to class and you sense resistance, you can offer that leaving at any time is always an option. It is important for someone to know they are not stuck. Giving someone this control has proven an effective way to decrease the anxiety of trying something new. A newcomer I had coaxed to class wrote in her evaluation, "I enjoyed this new yoga experience.

I never thought I would enjoy it. But I did, and it has been enjoyable. I feel relaxed and anxiety free."

**********

**To Recap:** Perhaps notice if Bessel van der Kolk's thoughts resonate more after this reading chapter on managing human dynamics:

> Social support is not the same as merely being in the presence of others. The critical issue is *reciprocity*: being truly heard and seen by other people around us, feeling that we are held in someone else's mind and heart.
>
> (van der Kolk, 2015)

I will note that his entire book is filled with similar insightful, compassionate, and inspiring ideas. Your challenge is to embrace your role as a classroom manager because you can create a room in which to build safety, to support empowerment, and to allow people to be heard and to be seen.

## References

Gordon, James. (2019). *The Transformation*. New York: Harper One.

Levine, Peter. (2010). *In an Unspoken Voice*. Berkeley, CA: North Atlantic Books.

Van der Kolk, Bessel A. (2015). *The Body Keeps the Score: Brain, Mind, and Body in the Healing of Trauma*. New York: Penguin Publishing, p. 79.

# 5
# For Teachers, Clinicians, and Health Care Providers

## Personal Qualities: Building a Sense of Safety

What's the number one consideration in personal qualities? It is still building a sense of safety. Trauma-informed yoga is not about summoning emotions and verbally exploring what it all means as you sit on a yoga mat. Trauma-informed yoga is about building feelings of safety so someone can experience and then learn to manage bodily sensations in a conscious and adaptive way. An inspiring thought from St. Augustine: "Since you cannot do good to all, you are to pay special attention to those who, by accidents of time, or place, or circumstance, are brought into closer connection to you." Let's look at personal qualities that can strengthen your ability both to build a sense of safety and to empower those who "are brought into closer connection to you."

### Dress for Success

Yep, appearances matter. We know that teachers in a yoga studio or health club may feel comfortable in more revealing attire. You do not want your words to distract or to trigger, so clothing choices should not either. Don't miss this trauma-informed opportunity. We can choose our words. We can choose our clothes. Once you find your trauma-informed style, the suggestion is to be consistent in how you dress. I had taught veterans for many years when one day there was a discussion of military uniforms. A veteran offered that I had a uniform – I always wore the same thing. Of course, he did not mean literally but the general pattern of dress. And he had noticed. 'Predictable and consistent'.

DOI: 10.4324/9781003308836-7

## Make Yourself Heard

Bessel van der Kolk, MD, said to a workshop of 300 people: "Yoga teachers may not realize the power they have … The quality of the voice can be a miraculous experience" (NICABM #2). Interestingly, he had asked and only two of us in attendance were yoga teachers. Why the voice is a primary gauge for safety is discussed in Chapter 1. Many ways to keep the thread of your voice going without causing the distractions of too much to process are outlined in Part II. But first, let's consider the personal qualities that contribute to the quality of your sound.

**Nature versus Nurture:** Typically, a female voice with its higher tones processed by the middle ear is more likely to signal safety. Low sounds signal danger. What if a teacher has a deep, low voice? Not being directive and observing other trauma-informed protocols can help capitalize on a positive quality of that low, deep voice: confidence. A deep voice using trauma-informed language in a confident tone can convey someone feels comfortable teaching. It can create a visceral *feeling* that this place is safe to practice making personal choices, to explore breathing and movement options, and to experience physical sensations and feelings. A principal in a low-income school, a long-time supporter of the GreenTREE classroom yoga break program, shared that a kindergartner told her he did the yoga breathing when his father beat him with a belt. In some way, the male yoga teacher's deep, confident voice had gone home with this little boy.

**A Thread to Safety:** We have discussed 'your voice is a thread to safety', but let's revisit the idea as part of your personal style. Do you teach in a stream-of-consciousness way, offering ideas and information based on what comes to your mind in the moment? Not wrong, but not trauma-informed. Your musings could be a voice leading someone astray, tangling the thread (to push the metaphor) by distracting from trauma-informed teaching opportunities. On the other hand, is it your style to leave periods of quiet? Again, not wrong, but not trauma-informed. Think of dead air on a radio station. You want people to stay tuned to your station. Perhaps envision your voice as a thread connecting you to others as it enables them to stay present. Ideas on how to keep that thread from getting tangled are in Chapter 9.

## Be Predictable and Consistent

**Stay Put:** Staying in one predictable spot while teaching shows respect for someone with strong startle reflexes. A hyperaware person may wonder if and when you might start circling looking for someone to correct. And if you say

"Eyes open, eyes closed, your choice," someone may not feel safe enough to explore that option.

**It's About Time:** Do you run late? This quality may be something you want to address. Part of being predictable is starting and ending the class on time. From my experience, if one person is present, start the class. If you wait, people tend to come later and later. Having extra mats already set out signals all are welcome. The suggestion is to end on time as well. If class ends at 3:00, plan so that you are done at 3:00, not starting the wrap-up. Again, don't miss an opportunity to create and to model consistent time boundaries.

**A Meet and Greet:** You can't teach this week – now what? One approach is to cancel class. However, I felt holding that space on Mondays was important so as not to break someone's weekly flow. Remembering the unease I had felt facing an unexpected substitute, I invited my sub to attend the week prior to meet everyone. I explained why I would be away. Interestingly, only one person chose not to come, emphatically saying, "If you are not here, I am not coming." Everyone else attended and eagerly shared how much they had enjoyed the new teacher. They chose to experience something new but within the safety of a known yoga class and a pre-approved teacher. 'Teach to Empower'.

**It's Still About Time:** We know that one way to support trauma recovery and to build resiliency skills is to look forward to something. My mother, who had experienced many years of complex trauma, used to say, "It's important to have a looking-forward-to." As I learned about trauma and the brain, I understood that her continued use of this phrase had enabled her to envision something good in the future so as not to feel stuck. Bessel van der Kolk talks about the importance of thinking about what happens next. All to say, if you offer to bring something next week, make sure you do. Someone asked while we were still standing in the hall, "Did you remember those new art things for the journals?" A most unlikely older veteran said to me, "I always look forward to what centerpiece you are going to bring. You should have been a florist." Take every opportunity to give someone a looking-forward-to. A refugee eagerly greeted me one week asking if I had remembered the extra rosemary. I had.

## Be Confident

Someone who sounds unsure and tentative does not inspire a feeling of safety. But being confident does not mean being directive and overbearing. Being confident means your trauma-informed suggestions can help someone feel safe enough to take their feelings of empowerment out for a spin. One way to gain that important sound of confidence in your voice is to practice. Some tried-and-true suggestions are in this chapter's last section.

**Meet You Poolside:** Part of completing the GreenTREE Yoga® certification program is taking a variety of yoga classes and writing observations. I had suggested a teacher to someone both with her own traumas and a commitment to teach trauma-informed yoga. As I read her observation, I was surprised to see the class had taken place outside by a recreation center pool. She only had wonderful things to say about the yoga experience. I attribute it to the warm, knowledgeable, and as importantly, confident teacher. These teacher qualities overrode all the potential triggers of a new place, a new teacher, and unpredictable distractions. Social engagement in action.

**A Quality Control Guy:** Be confident about what you are presenting. But also, be confident in yourself. We all make mistakes when we teach, which prompts Judith Hanson Lasater, PhD, to say in her workshops, "How human of me." You may forget one side of a sequence. Either you remember or someone reminds you. In my veterans' class, Joann has been my quality control person, and we still joke about it. I like that someone is paying attention. Someone said to me once, "I don't want to walk out lopsided."

Then, you have a choice as to how you respond. You can get flustered. Your group may feel your discomfort and feel now the yoga won't work, oh no. You can say, "Oh, let's go back and do that side now." Or "Okay, we will do it in reverse order on this side." You show you still have a plan. It's another opportunity to model moving through any feelings of discomfort with ease.

**Be All You Can Be:** As discussed in previous chapters, whether teaching short breaks or a full practice, you are a manager. A question arises. What should you do when you notice someone has shoulders slumped or appears collapsed? "If you like, gently press one shoulder back … Then press the other shoulder back." It's not directive but shows confidence in getting everyone set up for a better experience. Again, the trauma-informed suggestion is to teach to the group, not to identify someone in need of correction.

## Personal Challenges

### Learning to Stretch

I have a close friend who once said, "Yael, yoga is about stretching." As she is a gifted trauma therapist, I knew she did not mean stretching to touch my toes but rather stretching my window of tolerance. Her words echoed in my mind when someone asked me to take over the class at our men's state prison I offer this story to keep in the front of your teaching mind. Early on, the prison gave me many opportunities to stretch my comfort zone. To begin the story, I had never been in any prison. In the prison gym, I needed to face the door for my sense of safety. Stretch, yes. But know your stretching limits. Interestingly, I asked the guys how the previous two female teachers had set up: semicircle of mats, teacher facing the door. There is much to be learned and shared from The Prison Yoga Project's trauma-informed books for incarcerated people: *Yoga a Path for Healing and Recovery*, and *Freedom from the Inside, a Woman's Yoga Practice Guide* (www.prisonyoga.org). Now, back to my stretching practice.

**It's Cold in Here:** One day the guard asked if I wanted the heat on or off. When it was on, I had to raise my voice to be heard, which wasn't the effect I was going for. It got cold. A young man who was doing a yoga teacher training (kudos to Denise Druce at Yoga Assets for creating this program) mentioned to me after class that the older guys were cold and stiff. He had a solution. "We could pull the mats closer, so you don't have to shout." I weighed my strong need for personal space against the needs of the older, stiffer men. We huddled the mats closer. Yoga is about stretching. Thank you, Elizabeth!

**The Sweet Smell of Pine:** One more prison story. The woman who had taught the class previously had stocked a cabinet with essential oils. I thought, rather smugly I will admit, I will not use essential oils – not trauma-informed. Smell can be a potent trigger, and I had no idea what was going on in this group, other than I knew there probably was a high degree of trauma. I felt confident. No oils, not trauma-informed, not doing it. But that's not the story. Before 'Final Stretch', some of the guys explained the oils were in the back cabinet. So, I walked around the front of our semicircle, saying, "Lift your palm if you would like some oils." I put a few drops in a palm. Person after person rubbed the essences on their arms and faces, as if it were suntan oil. I also offered more on the way out. Later, the teacher who'd left the oil simply said, "Yes, they are starved for sensory stimulation." Lesson learned: have your guiding principles but know yoga is about stretching. Adapt as you gather more information about the considerations of your specific population.

**All Part of the Plan:** You may have the opportunity to stretch your class vision. In refugee or homeless or DV shelter classes, children can appear throughout what was supposed to be a practice for the older set. A teacher shared her thoughts with me.

> I helped them to connect with their kiddos and we worked together instead of it seeming like it was a negative distraction that children were there. When one of the children did a perfect child's pose (sitting up), I

acknowledged it and said, "I am not sure there is anything better than a little cutie doing child's pose." Some women were also holding their kids while doing some poses (even once they were doing downward dog with their little girl on their back). I acknowledged that as a sign of strength.

I have found children in a practice can create a wonderful dynamic. The focus shifts and creates a playful tone. The importance of play (*lila* in yoga philosophy) in expanding windows of tolerance is discussed on pages 24 and 144. Often adults, once they realize you welcome the children, will get more out of the practice. A trauma-informed teacher meets changes with flexibility, not annoyance.

## Self-care and Vicarious Trauma: Take Care of You

**'The Danger Has Passed':** In my trainings, I offer that taking care of yourself is not being selfish, it's being practical. The stress of being in a helping profession can take both a physical and emotional toll. If you become emotionally or physically unavailable, you are not as effective in your work. You may become someone who needs help. Increased levels of stress hormones help us rally to action to keep safe and to meet the demands of the situation. Yet, high levels of cortisol and adrenaline should subside when, as Winnie-the-Pooh says, "the danger has passed." Chapter 1 discusses how chronic stress can cause varying degrees of compromised immune function, anxiety, depression, pain, digestive problems, and sleep issues.

**The Three-legged Stool:** In 1975, Herbert Benson, MD, of Harvard Medical School, published a classic book called *The Relaxation Response*. It was one of the first to outline mind/body approaches to medicine in a time when self-care wasn't even in medical discussions. At that time, medical care was surgery and medications. In the updated book, Dr. Benson explains how he envisions a future in which medicine would "call upon self-care for 60-to-90 percent of the everyday problems patients experience" (Benson, 1975/1990/ 2000). He called medicine, surgery, and self-help a three-legged stool in which all legs are needed. His book outlines how someone can practice and learn responses that lower stress levels, lower heart rate, and lower blood pressure to promote health. As a cardiologist, he had the medical expertise to support his ideas. Let's look at more of the self-care leg of that stool.

**The Power of Laughter:** Why do many people like comedies? As mentioned, laughing is a long breath out and can lower stress levels in the body. Have you ever experienced nervous laughter? It seems another way the body releases stress. Perhaps compare the feelings of watching a comedy to those experienced while watching a holocaust or graphic war movie. Vicarious experiences cause secretions of many types of neurotransmitters. So, it makes physiological sense that working with people who have had traumas, even if you do not know the specifics, can affect you. Perhaps you are working with a group of survivors of torture, domestic abuse, or the sex trade. Again, even without the specifics, you can be affected by knowing some troubling events were experienced. You may even be retriggered from your own past traumas.

**Changing the Conversation:** Initially, job stress was referred to as job burnout. Typical advice was either to stop complaining or to get a new job. But then people committed to the issues started a conversation. The effects of job stress from contact with trauma, from working with people to animals to the environment, was named. Some attribute the term *compassion fatigue* to Carla Johnson, who in 1992 described what nurses experienced as the disconnection from their emotions from having to care for very ill patients (Johnson, 1992). Later, Charles Figley, PhD, aptly called compassion fatigue the cost of caring (Figley, 1995). Interestingly, the word compassion means suffering together. In his book *Born to Be Good: The Science of a Meaningful Life*, Dacher Keltner, PhD, discusses the ways in which our ability to respond to the cries and needs of others supports our species survival. Many religions, philosophers, and scientists write about this idea (Keltner, 2009). There is a clinical term for people who feel or care nothing for others: sociopaths.

Another term to describe the cost of caring is *vicarious trauma*, coined by Saakvitne and Pearlman (1996) to identify an actual change in one's world view. For example, a social worker may see a child at a toy store. The child has a large bruise on their arm, which causes the social worker to take a critical look at the parent and wonder what social services might be available. They are at a toy store: a shift in world view.

**I Said, "I'm Fine."** You may practice the personal mantra of "Oh, I am fine. I said I'm fine, okay". A 30-question PROQOL 5 survey can help assess how fine you are (see Appendix C: Supplemental Resources). The information can help to start a conversation with yourself. For clinicians and health care providers, the good news is that sharing a short yoga break can be a break for you too. As you teach a break to clients or patients, you are experiencing the benefits. But not so fast. If you feel unsure about teaching, if you rush, or if you feel stressed about if it's working, then it is not a break for anyone. If you are a yoga teacher working to teach in a more trauma-informed way, but you are feeling it's too many things to remember, then it's not part of your self-care. I offer that it doesn't matter if you are taking a trauma-informed class or teaching a class or a break, the benefits are there for you to experience. How can you make teaching part of your self-care program and not add to your work stress?

The last section of this chapter outlines simple, tried-and-true suggestions. One clinician shared he knew he was rushing his breaks, which made him feel anxious and he could hear it in his voice. "Moving forward, I'll want to pay close attention to this as I can imagine my elevated voice/nervous system might impede some of the benefits of trauma-informed yoga for my clients."

**Reframing in a Mindful Way:** Dr. Jack Kornfield's books on mindfulness discuss how to use self- awareness to your advantage (Kornfield, 1993, 2008). You notice you are rushing. Noticing, which is an observation in the present, is a first step in change. The next step is to decide what you want to do with the information. We can pull in an insight from Milton H. Erickson, MD, one which complements the mindfulness practice (Erickson, 1992). Once you have noticed something, you can reframe it, or consider it in a new way. Perhaps reframe your anxiety to "ah … an opportunity. A way to expand my repertoire. Let's see what I can do …" You can choose to reframe, or you sink in a mire of negative thoughts.

Two important resources for self-care are *The Compassion Fatigue Workbook: Creative Tools for Transforming Compassion Fatigue and Vicarious Traumatization* by Françoise Mathieu (2011) and *Trauma Stewardship: An Everyday Guide to Caring for Self While Caring for Others* by Laura van Dernoot Lipsky (2009). I have used these accessible resources in my self-care workshops for many years, and people find them easy-to-use and valuable.

Be nice to you. Set yourself up for success by knowing that becoming more trauma-informed is a process. A teacher told me he was not pleased with his teaching. "I was a little off this morning. Maybe I needed to get better sleep last night." I said the positive point was his awareness, which is a key step to change or to learning. Give yourself credit for noticing. Small steps signal success. Another teacher told me she spent the drive home from a class going over what she had done wrong. I told her, "You noticed. You did a lot right; I can tell from your notes. Be nice to you."

## Your Safety

Some well-intended staff may want to include yoga in their facility's program because they have heard yoga is a good thing. Yet yoga is not a magic wand with teachers as wizards. Referrals may come from therapists not familiar with yoga. You want to clarify who is a good fit for your class. Sample flyers are in Appendix C: Supplemental Resources. Once you have matched your class to participant needs, the next challenge is to identify available options to maintain both your own safety and your ability to teach.

**Is There a Plan B?** You may be teaching at a treatment facility, a shelter, a prison, a school, or a veterans' facility. Whether you are on staff or working as a consultant or volunteer, become familiar with the specific protocol for addressing issues. For example, someone may need immediate assistance outside your job description. One teacher told me well-intentioned treatment facility staff simply sent clients to do yoga. It was unfair both to her and to others in the class to expect her to address what were clearly non-yoga situations. A requested meeting with the director clarified the roles of the teacher and staff.

**Feel What You Feel:** One of my six weekly veterans' classes was in the evening in a locked building. It seemed fine at first. A class regular walked me to my car, which I truly appreciated as it was late. One class I found myself alone with a large male veteran I did not know, other than he was on his way to a residential treatment facility. Looking back, I saw how I had gone to extremes telling myself, "Oh, everything is fine. Don't think about it, no safety concerns here." Since no staff member was available to attend, I canceled my evening class in that lonely building.

**All Together Now:** If I am not 15 minutes early, I am late. So, I arrived at the state prison gym early. The hall guard, who knew more about the system than I did, invited me to wait in his office: "You might feel more comfortable here." He then hand-delivered me to the gym guard. The system then broke down a bit. Once during class, I looked up and didn't see the guard, who wandered back ten minutes later. There is a ten-minute window as the men move to the next class. Envision a small woman amid a sea of guys all leaving the gym and merging with others, without a guard in sight. Eventually, I spied some guards, all bunched up at the end of the long hall. Note to self: be aware of how things work in different systems. Your sense of safety counts too. I then timed my entrance and exit to meet the needs of my nervous system. I do want to note that the gym guard disappearing and reappearing did not bother me after the first class. I felt confident this group of very grateful and polite guys would keep me safe.

## What Are You Practicing?

It is called a yoga practice because we are always practicing. As we refine our teaching, a reasonable question becomes, "What are you practicing?" In what ways are you practicing "Know thyself," the wise words of Socrates?

**Clear Intentions:** Again, a question to continually ask is: "Does what I am doing and what I am saying meet my intention of sharing yoga in a trauma-informed way?" It also is worth reminding yourself that your role is as a guide, a role embraced by many leading trauma therapists. A yoga perspective from the foundational teacher T.K.V. Desikachar is a guru "is not one who says, 'I am the guru' ... One of the qualities of a person who is clear, who is wise, is not to need to say 'I am clear, I am wise'" (Desikachar, 1999).

A therapist who teaches 30-minute yoga practices with his refugee clients shared: "I have had breakthroughs in my personal yoga practice that the yoga teacher had no idea about. I think many therapists get into the false notion that our clients are not as smart as we are and can't figure things out without us being there to intervene with our specially trained interventions." Included in this astute comment is the same message to yoga teachers. Trust with your trauma-informed guidance, someone can find their way.

**'Stay in Your Lane':** I have observed one of the greatest challenges for clinicians, health care providers, and teachers is to 'Stay in Your Lane'. Many have shared the image of 'Stay in Your Lane' as helpful during short yoga breaks in a clinical session. It is a total lane switch. Part of trauma-informed protocols includes resisting the desire or habit to explain first and later deconstruct what you did. A clinician in my training shared that after he did a yoga break, he suggested a list of ways for the client to compare and contrast the breathwork. He told me he thought, "Huh, that felt very therapist of me. I may be undoing the sensory experience with too many words. It's definitely tricky for me to stay in my lane. I want to practice more as I move forward."

Yet the 'Stay in Your Lane' also applies to yoga teachers. The challenge is to avoid weaving a bit of talk therapy into the yoga. Several thoughtful and caring yoga teachers have asked if they should have a new student intake questionnaire. That's an unequivocal no. Again, trauma-informed doesn't mean you are informed about someone's trauma. It means you are informed about protocols to support trauma recovery and to build resiliency skills. For both the clinician and the teacher, 'Stay in Your Lane' can be a useful mantra. Perhaps think of it as keeping what you are offering undiluted. It's pure yoga, whether a short break or a full practice. Again, it becomes self-care for you too.

**Old Dog, New Tricks:** Language plays a major role in how we do what we do. In my experience, identifying and practicing your own trauma-informed way of using language is another big challenge for teachers, clinicians, and health care providers. A therapist told me, "My training as a clinician has brought a heavy focus on the verbal. Shifting away from this will take some time but will be a welcomed change as I add trauma-informed yoga breaks into therapy sessions." A teacher told me, "I really need to work on my choice of words. I find myself saying relax." For part-time yoga teachers, the verbal skills from their other jobs can easily creep in. A lawyer, used to justifying everything, or a businessperson, used to pitching new ideas, is challenged with reworking how they communicate. Awareness is the first step. Simplifying all you know into a body-based, empowering instruction is a challenge. But the result is a stronger trauma-informed program, making it well worth the effort.

**It's Not About You:** There are some yoga situations in which it is appropriate for the instructors to focus their energies on what they can demonstrate to their full yogic abilities without much awareness of others. Trauma-informed yoga is not that situation. Or quite simply, it is not about you. Hanging out in an advanced king dancer because it is, after all, your favorite pose, may prove frustrating to others. A teacher shared an observation. "I also need to keep my eyes open! Ugh! I know it's not my practice, but I feel that yoga feeling come over me too as the teacher and the next thing I know, I've closed my eyes."

Another point to consider is the class is not about your feelings of frustration, irritation, or disappointments of the day. A trauma-informed approach is to check your emotional baggage at the door. Make that part of your practice, and it's a win for everyone as the yoga practice can improve your day as well. Chapter 4 discusses the importance of managing people in the room who might be triggering to others. You and your troubles can be triggering as well. So a gentle reminder: it's not about you.

**It Is About You:** If you want to grow your yoga teaching, grow your personal practice. The more yoga you experience, the more your repertoire grows. I keep a notebook of the new poses/flows that I like from other classes. I might be inspired to incorporate a trauma-informed variation. I am not one who journals but keeping a simple list allows me to grow as a teacher. Noting what you like is helpful. Yet noting what you do not like can be as instructive. Notice your feelings: calm, discomfort, safety, being judged, anxiety, connection to the group. Then notice what elicited these feelings: the space, the breathwork, the language, the music, the poses, the teacher, others in the room.

**Different Dance Steps:** Some can be thrown if there are differing abilities in a class. But, if you teach to empower, someone can find what they need and notice themselves more in the process. Someone can focus on how the simple breathwork and movement feel, not on what you showed as the right way to do it. Accepting your role as a guide takes pressure off you. You no longer have to model every variation or to try to match everyone's breathing patterns. Consider you are successful if someone chooses to take a seat and explore 'what feels like a comfortable stretch to you today'.

## 'You Need Yoga'

**Responsible Referrals:** In a trauma-informed setting, there is more to being responsible than being on time. Some make unsubstantiated claims about how yoga cures all. There may be compelling physical or psychological reasons why someone needs medication or to limit movement. An offhand comment of 'you need yoga' can miss the mark. Yes, yoga as an art and science has been around for thousands of years, bringing mind, body, and breath together for health and healing. But do you mean Ashtanga, Vinyasa, Hatha, Kundalini, Yin, power, or restorative yoga? Do you mean laughter, hot, aerial, partner, naked, or goat yoga? Do you mean yoga in a fitness center, a local library, a yoga studio, someone's meadow, or a private class? Do you mean yoga taught by a fitness-oriented teacher, a meditation teacher, a teacher who plays loud rock music, or someone who thought teaching yoga would be fun to try? Each is a real option. You may be grasping the idea that not only are there many yoga styles, but there are many types of yoga teachers and many settings in which to teach. Some teachers fancy themselves as gurus who know all, some as guides, and some haven't given it much thought.

Before my trauma-informed days when teaching at a fitness center, someone arrived at the yoga room and said, and I quote, "I just had back surgery. My doctor said I needed to do yoga." I suggested perhaps they get more information about what kind of yoga, and I respectfully sent them away.

**Set Up for Success:** Let's look at how you can consider available yoga options. A more fit person may need an athletic, pound-it-out style to reconnect with themselves. I know people with multiple traumas who started their yoga experiences with hot yoga or Ashtanga, both yoga styles with challenging poses in a prescribed (predictable and consistent) order. Then later they preferred something different, a Hatha or Vinyasa (flow) class.

- **Empower.** What started as a one-page handout to find a trauma-informed class grew to two pages as more information was requested (Appendix C: Supplemental Resources). One suggestion is simply: "You can leave a class anytime you feel uncomfortable or unsafe." I realized how much this option was needed as people continue to say, "Really, I can just leave?"

- **Ask teachers.** You may know yoga teachers who can make suggestions as to classes or teachers that might be a good fit.
- **Proceed with caution.** You can read class descriptions on yoga websites and read about the teachers. But a name doesn't make it so. Some well-intended yet uninformed teachers and yoga studios put trauma-informed in a class name when the class and teacher are not. With remote classes more accessible, there is no shortage of trauma-informed class names. Empower someone to leave a room or to disconnect from a class that is making them *feel* unsafe for any reason.
- **Proceed with more caution.** Certain styles of yoga can appear trauma-informed. A restorative yoga class usually consists of lying still for five to ten minutes, sometimes in quiet. Neither lying still nor being in quiet is trauma-informed. A yin class is holding stretches for several minutes, again there may not be enough physical movement to make it trauma-informed. We circle back to this idea in Chapter 8.

## 'Trust the Yoga'

'Trust the Yoga' also can be a personal challenge. Again (and again) yoga has been practiced for thousands of years because it works.

**Smile for the Camera – Remote Classes:** Teaching remotely and providing telehealth clinical services allow expanded access to many services. For yoga teachers, it has become a time in which to 'Trust the Yoga', as we can be teaching to an audience of one – ourselves on the screen. When I had to change my classes to remote, I was surprised when a long-time student offered that she was glad I felt more comfortable teaching. She said, "I can tell because you don't sound nervous anymore." Not being able to see my students was a real challenge, but in the end, it strengthened my efforts to empower people to find what they needed today.

A teacher shared the challenge of teaching in-person and on-screen at the same time. "I need be more aware of when my heart rate goes up so I can take a few breaths immediately before proceeding. Because I didn't take a sec to notice myself, the pacing was a bit quicker than I would have liked." Indeed, it is challenging to teach in-person and on-screen. One class I taught had veterans in the room with me and three telehealth locations on one screen. I also had one veteran on the phone. Thursdays at one had a bit of a yoga party feel. While you can 'Trust the Yoga', it's not a blind trust. You may need to iterate the process to find ways to make everyone *feel* comfortable, safe, and included. The suggestion is to make refining your trauma-informed skills part of *your* practice.

Finding ways to connect is key. A few times during class, I address a group or person I know. I include the person on the phone. For example, I might say, "Alex, how is the air in Pocatello today?" Or, "Ben, did you do the Costco stretch this week?" as he had explained it to us last week. To end the class, I might say, "Well, Sam, if you are ever at our VA, stop by so we can share some carrot cake." It is about finding a balance. You want to create a connection, but you do not want to create a distraction. Refining your trauma-informed ways to connect with your group can build teaching confidence. In case you are wondering, to practice the Costco stretch rest your heel on the floor, press your foot against the wheel on a grocery cart, and pull your toes toward your shin. Keeping a slight bend in that knee protects the knee joint. Repeat on the other side.

**Think Before You Leap:** A teacher working with a grief and loss clinician met with a group whose husbands had recently committed suicide. To introduce balance poses, she asked if something had thrown them off balance recently. You may have just gasped. Yes, she too immediately knew it was the wrong thing to say. She quickly moved on to the balance poses and breathwork, without doing the visualization she had planned. She asked me what she should have done. I thought she handled it well. Focus on the body-based approach. Be flexible as needed. She learned she needed to be more aware of what she had planned for grief and loss groups.

I have my own story. As I have mentioned, before my trauma-informed days, I taught at a fitness center. A young woman unexpectedly brought her mom to my 90-minute class. For 'Final Stretch', I sometimes would recite a memorized poem that supported the day's body-based meditation. This day it was Elizabeth Coatsworth's "There are rivers that I know, borne of ice and melting snow …" which provided opportunities for guided imagery. Halfway through the recitation, I froze and wanted to go through the floor, literally. After the practice, a regular participant said, "What happened? I have never heard you stumble." What had happened was that as I was talking about "rivers borne of ice and melting snow, white with rapids, swift to roar," I remembered that last year this woman's 16-year-old son had drowned in such a river in our nearby canyon. But I pressed on and quickly finished. After class, the woman approached me, and I braced. She smiled warmly at me and said it was a wonderful class, just what she had needed. 'Trust the Yoga'.

**A Multi-use Tool:** 'Trust the Yoga' has many applications. Yet another is trust that it works for you as well. I found myself sitting in a circle of male veterans

I did not know who had walked from the residential treatment center. I had taught many different groups, but I sat there unable to speak. One guy was on his mat doing pushups. I wondered what I could offer that would be of interest to these men. The seconds ticked by into a minute of quiet and more doubt. I remember thinking, "If you don't speak now, you are not going to be able to. Say something, anything." I started teaching what I knew. And it was a fine class based on their comments. This experience gave me confidence when I headed to the state prison. I had more opportunities to trust that teaching the yoga would calm me as I taught. It did, every time.

## Trust Yourself

You bring a wonderful and key ingredient to your teaching – yourself. The suggestion is to run your ideas through the trauma-informed filter: building safety, supporting empowerment, and maintaining simplicity. Again, ask, "Does what I am saying and what I am doing meet my intention of teaching in a trauma-informed way?" Then make it your own. I think we have all experienced the value of authentic teaching as opposed to a more perfunctory style. Something will occur to me. I run it through my trauma-informed filter. I try it. I gauge the response. This process over many years is how the phrases in Tables 11.1, 11.2, and 11.3 came to be. Let's look to some teachers and clinicians for more examples.

**To Meet or Not to Meet?** A yoga teacher in a residential facility was scheduled for an individual session. The woman arrived, clearly agitated from therapy. "I didn't ask if she were okay or what was wrong when I first went to pull her for a session, I simply asked, 'Would you still like to meet today?' I just figured it wasn't my place and, if she needed to process something it should be with her therapist, unless she felt like she wanted/needed to share with me. So, my question is, how would you approach that situation?" I told her I thought she handled it well. She gave the client total control. The woman probably needed to get out of the language part of her brain and in touch with her physical self. After the trauma-informed yoga practice, the teacher wrote, "I am really glad I listened to my teacher's intuition."

**Checking In:** Another teacher shared that someone left class, and she saw them later. Should she approach them and check in or just give them space? She trusted that she needed to give it more thought. I suggested she could offer, "I noticed you left our Wednesday practice. Is there a question maybe I could help with? Perhaps come another time, and again, you can leave anytime if it's not a good fit for that day." 'Teach to Empower'.

**Setting the Stage:** A clinician told me that he was teaching a 30-minute class to refugee women. He felt setting a boundary of a few minutes at the beginning of class to listen to their stories created a relationship, a point from which he could then teach the class. I had confidence that this warm and talented clinician using those few minutes to establish that personal connection was a good choice. I use 'Opening Connections', to begin a refugee class (p. 179). A note of caution: inviting open-ended sharing can create triggering situations. Know your group. 'Opening Connections' creates connections by sharing food and yoga stories.

**When You Are Ready:** A teacher shared that someone arrived quite escalated. She gave the woman two minutes to vent because it was a private class. "I simply nodded and said, 'Sounds like you have a lot going on. When you are ready, shift forward on your feet …' and we got started with the class." Another example of trusting yourself. She created a window for the woman to connect and to be heard but moved quickly to the practice, using simple breathwork and movement to ground. 'Show, Don't Tell'.

**Rock On:** A treatment facility rule was no client music. A woman wanted to play her music in her individual session. The teacher explained that if any lyrics were inappropriate, they would have to skip the song. The woman agreed. The teacher's flexibility allowed the woman to feel some control as she used her music to create connections. I suggested the teacher ask if another time they could play music for 15 minutes, then play no music for 15 minutes and notice how that felt. If she said no, that was fine too. 'Teach to Empower'.

**So, Trust Yourself:** Rachel Naomi Remen, MD, has devoted her life to helping people heal from trauma and vicarious trauma. I share one full page from her book *Kitchen Table Wisdom* in my trauma trainings. "Expertise cures, but wounded people can best be healed by other wounded people … only other wounded people can understand what is needed, for the healing of suffering is compassion, not expertise" (Remen, 1996). Trust yourself to know when practicing simple breathwork, a grounding pose, or an energizing flow could provide benefits. Let's look at some ideas to seamlessly incorporate short ways to help someone practice ways to self-regulate.

## Ways to Incorporate Yoga into All You Do

The following chapters offer many ways to do simple breathwork and short movement breaks, but let's get a quick preview with a clinical backdrop. Why are the reasons for using a short yoga break in a clinical setting or in a yoga class the same? The short answer is you can teach these breaks in any setting when you notice someone would benefit from changing their affect state, that is, practicing self-regulation tools. Please note, yes again, it is trauma-informed to teach to the group, not to single someone out. Everyone can benefit from practicing. And now for the longer answer.

## On Your Mark, Get Set ...

**To begin** a yoga practice or a clinical session, a short break can provide ways to ground or to energize. It can provide tools to change a physiological state, either up-regulating or down-regulating. Quite simply, someone can perk up or calm down. This ability to self-regulate is a key to how someone processes what is happening. These ideas are at the core of Stephen Porges' polyvagal theory discussed in Chapter 1. I used to close a four-hour workshop with a one-hour 'Yoga for You' practice. But once I started with that practice. I noticed I had a markedly different group, much less stressed and more open to learning. People continue to comment that what they noticed was how stressed they were when they arrived, yet how they now felt calmer, how they became aware of the fact they weren't breathing, and how they were able to slow down and notice how the stretches felt. A health care or clinical session isn't four hours, but it could be one or two hours.

**In the middle** of a class or session, you notice someone appears collapsed, disconnected, or agitated. Working with the cues presented in the body works around language limitations. The well-placed yoga break can help someone to interrupt their stress cycle, to move out of a collapsed state, or to become less agitated. The break can help someone re-engage with what you are offering. A well-placed yoga break can help someone get unstuck by becoming more grounded in the present.

> ... Your hand opens and closes / And opens and closes. / If it were always a first / Or always stretched open, / You would be paralyzed. / Your deepest presence is in every small / Contracting and expanding. / The two as beautifully balanced and coordinated /
> As bird wings. ~ Rumi (1207–1273)

Pairing a breath in with a simple opening movement and pairing a breath out with a simple closing movement can create, and then reinforce, a visceral feeling of not being stuck. Two examples, and there are many in this book, include tree pose and a standing flow.

- **Tree Pose:** "When you are ready, stand in a way that makes you feel strong today. One hand may be on the chair. If you like, put one or both hands over your heart. The suggestion is to practice 3 breaths. As you breathe in, arm(s) open, fingers stretch wide. As YOU breathe out, hand(s) over your heart." (*Say 3 times slowly.*)

- **Seated/Standing Flow:** "The suggestion is to practice 3 breaths. Longer breaths in *can* be energizing. As YOU breathe in, look up and stretch up, fingertips press overhead. As YOU breathe out, arms release, *fingertips* tap on legs." (*Say 3 times slowly.*)

**To end** on a positive note, a yoga break gives someone the opportunity to *feel* some bodily sensations after what may have been a useful but stressful talking session. For example, 'Goal Post Breathing' provides grounding through breathwork paired with arm movements (p. 132). Practicing a self-regulation technique at the session's end also is an opportunity to set a two-minute plan to use later in the day or night when someone wants to change how they are feeling. The suggestion is to offer one new break a session, providing support with a handout, an MP3 and an MP4 of that one break (Appendix C: Supplemental Resources). 'More is not better, more is confusing'.

## Use as Needed

**Give It a Rest:** Talk therapy can be a wonderful and important tool for trauma recovery, but it can also be challenging for someone not fully engaged with the language part of the brain. A short break as needed can give that part of the brain a rest. A therapist shared with me that, "They don't realize how much we are doing in a short yoga flow. People expect talking, so it doesn't interrupt their expectations. Even though the talk is about the sensorimotor system and not the trauma narrative or other cognitively based things. I hesitate to use the word sneaky, but folks don't realize how much therapy they are doing when just moving and breathing."

A short break added by an astute health care provider, clinician, or teacher can raise a stress threshold or widen someone's window of tolerance. Someone may think or *feel*: "Oh, okay, stressful talking happening, stressful feelings happening." Enter the two-to-five-minute break (p. 190) with you as the safe guide. Someone then may think or *feel*: "Oh, okay, I can breathe and move through these feelings of discomfort." A therapist told me a client shared at the session's end, "This was less intense than previous sessions." It hadn't been, but he had included some breaks. Another client said, "I appreciate the break from the other work we are doing." A helpful tool to teach is the one-minute 'Anytime, Anywhere Breath' (p. 130).

**Get Organized:** A change of body position can calm someone in the present. A therapist offered this break to an extremely triggered woman in a group therapy session. A veteran had become so abusive that she had to be removed from the room by veterans' police. This story was relayed to me as both women attended my classes. The triggered woman said the therapist had taken her into the quiet hall. She stood against a wall, doing eagle pose and breathing with the therapist. They did not talk about what had happened or what eagle pose was supposed to do. Eagle pose does what Bessel van der Kolk says he likes about yoga: "it organizes the attentional system" (NICABM #2). She said it made her feel calmer and able to return to the session. The therapist was trained in trauma-informed yoga. 'Show, Don't Tell'.

## Ways to 'Practice What You Teach'

Why practice? Singers take voice lessons. The useful takeaway is someone can learn to use their voice in new ways. Again, the more you practice, the more comfortable and confident you can feel and therefore sound. Then teaching becomes a break for you as well.

**Get Ready, Get Set ...** Using the scripts as written is a strong starting point (Appendix A). At first glance, you may find the scripts repetitive, which they are, and lacking imagery, which is by design. But consider these comments echoed in many observations from yoga teachers and clinicians who practiced the GreenTREE Yoga® scripts.

1) **Simplicity:** The scripts are written simply, easy to use, and therefore easy to memorize or adapt.

   - **From a clinician:** "The script was very simple, I am not always a big fan of following a script, but this was really easy to read and to lead at the same time, I really like the simple, easy cues and the YOU breathe in. Very personal. It made me feel seen. It made me feel seen and that is so important for everyone, especially those with trauma." ~ M.L.
   - **From a yoga teacher:** "I love the simple words. I have tried to write out my own scripts, but I must make them too complicated because I can't read 'em. So, I love this." ~ M.B.

2) **Rhythmicity:** People like the rhythm of the phrases. The rhythm is like a poem and decreases their stress while they teach.

   - **From a clinician:** "The scripts are like poems – that's the feeling I got as I read them." ~ J.W.

3) **Awareness:** Both teachers and clinicians realize they tend to add extra words to share what they know. The suggestion is to first read the scripts as written so you can experience that extra words are just that – extra. 'More is not better, more is confusing'.

- **From a yoga teacher:** "I love the teaching. It's concise, there is repetition, and I love that it's YOU, as YOU breathe in, coming back to that in so many ways. I guess I didn't think of it, how important it was." ~ D.S.
- **From a therapist:** "I like the emphasis on YOU, the empowering part of the script. I found reading the script relaxing and I felt the nice slow pace. When I teach, I feel rushed - I have so much I want to say. It felt really good to slow down and teach in a more deliberate way." ~ J.P.

## Do Try This at Home

Let's look at simple ways to practice. Again (and again), the suggestion is to practice the scripts exactly as written at first. Then you can make it your own by following the basic principles of a trauma-informed approach: building safety, supporting empowerment, and maintaining simplicity.

1. **Choose one break to practice:**
   - Read the short break aloud twice.
   - Record an audio as you read the break. There are free recording apps for both phones and computers.
   - Listen to the audio. Note such things as if you are talking too quickly, too slowly, in a sing-song, or if you couldn't help putting in extra words (quite common). Again, you should sound like the authentic you.
   - Record it again as you both read and practice the break.
   - Then play the break and practice along with your recording. Was it too fast? Too slow? Would it be helpful to repeat this step?

2. **Take it out for a spin:**
   - Invite someone (coworker, friend, family) to practice the audio break with you.
   - Ask for comments (verbal or written). Keep recording until you hit your target points: confidence, simplicity, and sounding like yourself. A teacher told me she practiced with family. They thought it was too slow. Her written comment to me: "Oh, well (shrug)." I would offer that is not practicing in the spirit of being trauma-informed.

3. **Step it up:** Repeat the above steps using two or more breaks.

**********

**To Recap:** How you dress, how you sound, how you manage the space and people in that space, and your personal qualities all contribute to the effectiveness of your teaching. Being aware of your personal challenges as you hone your trauma-informed skills is a critical part of developing a more effective style. Practicing what you teach and how you teach *before* you teach will allow you to become more flexible and confident. You are therefore more able to build a sense of safety, to support empowerment, and to maintain simplicity.

## References

Benson, Herbert. (1975/1990/2000). *The Relaxation Response.* New York: William Morrow, p. XLII.

Desikachar, T. K. V. (1999). The Heart of Yoga: Developing a Personal Practice. Rochester, VT: Inner Traditions, p. XXVII.

Erikson, Milton. (1992). *Creative Choice in Hypnosis.* New York: Irvington Publishers, pp. 105; 216–217.

Figley, C. R. (1995). Compassion Fatigue: Toward a New Understanding of the Costs of Caring. In *Secondary Traumatic Stress: Self-Care Issues for Clinicians, Researchers, and Educators,* ed. B. H. Stamm. New Britain, CT: The Sidran Press, pp. 3–28.

Johnson, Carla. (1992). Coping and Compassion Fatigue. *Nursing,* 22(4), 116–121.

Keltner, Dacher. (2009). *Born to Be Good: The Science of a Meaningful Life.* New York: W. W. Norton and Company.

Kornfield, Jack. (1993). *A Path with Heart.* New York: Bantam Books.

Kornfield, Jack. (2008). *The Wise Heart.* New York: Bantam Books.

NICABM #2. *When Mindfulness Will (and Won't) Work for Treating Trauma with Bessel van der Kolk, MD.*

Remen, Rachel. (1996). *Kitchen Table Wisdom.* New York: Riverhead Books, p. 217.

Saakvitne, K. W., et al. (1996). *Transforming the Pain: A Workbook on Vicarious Traumatization.* New York: W. W. Norton and Company.

# PART II
# Teaching Protocols

# 6
# The Breath
## Considerations

---

Breathing, as you know from experience, is personal. T.K.V. Desikachar taught that the first step in a yoga practice is to link breath and body. He also wrote: "The breath should be your teacher" (Desikachar, 1995/1999). Or quite simply, notice how you are breathing and learn from that. Is your breathing quick and shallow, labored, strong and steady, or even happening? Okay, you notice and then what? Then you can manage your breath. How you breathe is something over which you can have conscious control. How you breathe directly affects your heart rate, blood pressure, and muscle tension. Some share that they had not realized they were holding their breath before we did breathwork. You may think, "Ah – these people would benefit from detailed directions on how to breathe to feel better." While at times this approach may be useful, it is instructive to note that B.K.S. Iyengar wrote that for some breathwork (pranayama) could be very agitating.

Let's consider how a prescribed breathing pattern, or telling someone how they should breathe, can be triggering. "Breathe in for five counts, pause for five counts, breathe out for eight counts, then pause for five counts." The breathing pattern may not be a good option for someone today. Yet they may feel compelled to do it, not wanting to displease you or to feel as though they have failed at one more thing. We know that for some a longer breath out can be triggering. Soldiers are taught to fire on the long breath out, which makes sense as that breath can lower heart rate and lower blood pressure. One veteran in my class told me her husband, deployed three times as a sniper in Afghanistan, flat out refused to do any of the breathing she had tried to share at home.

This chapter outlines *why* a trauma-informed approach to teaching simple breathwork builds safety, supports empowerment, and maintains simplicity. Because there is not one specific breath for raising stress thresholds or one specific breath to ground, Chapter 7 outlines *how* to teach a variety of

DOI: 10.4324/9781003308836-9

trauma-informed breathwork. Again, the ideas are a place to start with firm footing, a place from which to grow your program as meets your personal and professional goals. 'Be informed and be inspired'.

## Building Safety

If, as Stephen Porges, PhD, and other experts tell us, a trauma recovery priority is building a feeling of safety, it starts with the individual. If someone's heart is racing and their breathing is labored, they may not be feeling safe in their bodies. Dr. Porges explains when someone is stressed, their physiological resources are diverted to addressing these threats, again real or perceived. Diverted resources, which include your attention and your energy, mean you cannot fully engage in trauma recovery or building resiliency skills (Porges, 2011).

## A Key to Self-regulation

Why is it adaptive to practice breathwork to self-regulate? We can experience how it *feels* to manage our breathing. We can pause and then respond using the thinking (cortical) brain, rather than being trapped in the emotionally reactive or survival (subcortical) brain. Or quite simply, we can become more proactive and less reactive. Note that the phrase is self-regulation, which means someone is regulating their responses. Being told what to do and how it will feel is following directions, not self-regulating.

All of which again brings us back to the main and most inspiring point. Experts tell us that managing how we breathe is a conscious way we can manage our physiological state. How we breathe can lower heart rate, lower blood pressure, and lower muscle tension in real-time.

**A Path to Feeling:** To practice self-regulation, someone first must notice they are feeling physical, emotional, or mental discomfort, stress, collapse, or even despair. Yet someone who has experienced trauma may have reduced interoception, the ability to notice bodily sensations and to feel and verbalize emotional states (aspects of dissociation and alexithymia). What does this have to do with breathing? Simple breathwork can be a path to reconnecting with these sensations: that is, a path to feeling.

**A Path to Thinking:** High levels of stress hormones drive reactive emotional and instinctive (subcortical) responses, that is, no thought required. These responses can be adaptive as quick survival responses. As a veteran noted in an article on veterans' suicide, "Something happens over there … You wake up a primal part of your brain you are not supposed to listen to and it becomes a part of you …" (Phillipps, 2015). Physiological triggers can prove maladaptive over time. Simple breathwork can lower stress. Simple breathwork can support a path to thinking, which literally takes more time than survival or emotional responses.

**A Path to Learning:** As discussed in Chapter 1, sustained elevated stress levels can decrease someone's ability to learn. Learning happens as you pay attention. While most people are not trying to learn quantum physics, they may be rebuilding their lives by going to school, honing a new skill, or learning new responses to triggering stimuli. Being able to use breathwork to self-regulate empowers someone to widen their window of tolerance. 'It's body physiology'. In that way, breathwork becomes a path to learning.

**Begin at the Beginning:** Does it matter if you cue the breath or the movement first? You decide. If you like, read this cue slowly as you practice it. "Stretch your arms overhead and breathe in. When you are ready, release your arms and breathe out." Now, if you like, read this cue slowly as you practice it. "As YOU breathe in, arms stretch overhead. As YOU breathe out, arms release." Did it feel the same? Maybe it did, but many have shared that beginning with the breath had a smoother feel. Perhaps try it again. Consider that starting with the breath puts the breath in its rightful place: front and center in all things yoga. If the breath can support all these paths to healing, it makes sense to begin at the beginning.

## Grounding to Building Body Awareness

A veteran wrote after my class: "I can finally feel by breathing. I could not before. It feels really good." As a health care provider, clinician, or teacher, where do you start? With clear and simple guidance, you can help someone experience the feeling of being in the present using something that is always available: their breath. "Perhaps notice if you are breathing in through your nose," or "When you notice you are breathing … when you notice you are breathing, wiggle your fingers," can only be done in the present.

**Adding the Body – Movement and Proprioception:** Pairing breathwork with movement gives someone visual and tactile sensory cues they are not stuck. We know movement can reduce stress, so linking breathwork with movement in a clear way can prevent the distraction of someone wondering if they are breathing right. We know that trauma can compromise the part of the brain involved in proprioception, or awareness of where the body is in space. Body movements someone can both see and feel can help reactivate those neural pathways. "As I breathe in, I can see and feel that my fingers are stretching wide." Or "As I breathe in, I can see and feel my arm arcing over my head."

**Adding the Body's Largest Organ – Skin and the Sense of Touch:** The fact that the hands and the feet are physical areas with high concentrations of touch receptors can be used to your teaching advantage. Note that the cue stays simple so as not to distract from noticing sensations. "As YOU breathe in, toes press (or hands or fingertips or palms) … As YOU breathe out, release." Someone may notice rough palms, a cushiony mat, a soft fabric, or a cool metal chair. But again you are not giving a laundry list of choices. They notice what they notice. Pressing against a wall or one's leg can increase the degree of touch sensation. I worked with a young teen, an adoptee with a lifetime of traumas. She liked practicing breathwork with her hand on her trusted dog.

## Potential Breathing Triggers

**Why Words Matter:** It is no challenge to think of words or phrases that might be trauma triggers. Blow, lips, and thighs are examples. Examples include blow out through your lips or blow out a loud, fiery breath. Someone who works with sex trade survivors shared they are told to just take deep breaths out. You can understand how this well-intended breathwork cue could elicit a stress response. Finding the right phrase can be an iterative process, but one that keeps us mentally engaged. I used to say, "Breathe out as if you are blowing out a candle." I finally realized that type of breath could be fast and loud and triggering. What do you notice as you practice this revised cue? "If you like, practice a longer breath in … When you are ready, breathe out as if through a straw." That simple cue creates sensations without mention of mouths or pursed lips or rates of speed.

**So Many Breaths:** As with postures having vulnerable head or hip positions, some breathwork may be triggering to those new to yoga or early in their trauma recovery process. Various forms of extreme or loud breathwork may be better introduced much later (meaning after months or years, not later in the class) or not at all. James Nestor's book, *Breath: The New Science of a Lost Art* (2020) provides an engaging history of how breathwork has been used across time and cultures. It also presents interesting science on the effects of many breathing protocols. Certainly, prescribed breathing patterns can benefit some. But a trauma-informed approach to breathwork avoids these potentially triggering breaths.

- **Complicated breathing patterns** can be distracting to a brain in which the language centers are not in full use or in which pain or sleep challenges cause mental fatigue.
- **Constricted breaths** (sandbag on chest or yoga strap around back) can increase anxiety. I attended a workshop in which a nationally known presenter insisted we all put sandbags on our chests. I assume to build breath awareness. She got visibly irritated when I would not continue with what to me was an agitating exercise. She insisted it was wonderful. I felt as though I were fighting with my breath.
- **Noisy breaths** with loud breathing or panting (bellows or ujjayi) from yourself or others can cause discomfort or even feelings of panic.
- **Prescribed counting** provides structure (e.g. four-square breath), but it does not allow someone to explore a breathing pattern to manage their present state of arousal (or lack of). Science tells us there is a physiological response to the length of the breaths and to pauses. Prescribed breathing patterns can work against self-regulation and instead heighten an unwanted feeling state with no tools to manage those feelings and emotions.
- **Sustained longer breaths in** can build body heat or increase $CO_2$ levels in the body, causing feelings of anxiety.
- **Affect-shifting breaths** causing sudden changes in feeling states can signal an out-of-control feeling (e.g. Tummo or Wim Hof breathing).

**'It's Body Physiology':** An interesting science note is why feeling as though you can't breathe can cause stress responses. There is a subcortical part of the brain, unrelated to the amygdala (the fear center) and completely outside of conscious control, that feeds physiologic alarms when someone feels they are suffocating. Again, it is an automatic, physiologic response, unrelated to emotion and set off by increased carbon dioxide levels in the blood.

## 'Your Voice Is a Thread to Safety'

Much discussion has been given to how a voice can activate the social engagement system. How do we continue this thread to safety in breathwork practices?

**Do Breathwork and Talking Mix?** Consider that you are listening to a radio station, and it becomes dead air. First, you may think, "What happened, is everything okay? Is this a test or maybe an actual emergency?" You may change the station. Or you may wait, but in the ensuing silence you start thinking about something else. Consider that when you stop talking, you are taking away 'your voice as a thread to safety'. Even someone not listening to your words can tell by your tone that you feel safe. All is well.

**Dead Air Is Dead Air:** But isn't breathwork more effective when it's quiet? Well, dead air is still dead air: the thread (the connection) has been lost. Someone with trauma has, as Bessel Van der Kolk says, "lost their way in the world" (van der Kolk, 2015). Why? Many disconnections have happened: among signals in the brain, from bodily and emotional sensations, with personal relationships, and to community ties. You can use your trauma-informed skills to empower someone to reconnect with their breath, with their body, and with others. "Now, take five deep breaths and you will feel better," and then waiting for a minute in quiet is not only directive but could increase feelings of disconnection. Is it better to say, "If you like, practice five breaths in any way that feels comfortable to you today," and then wait in quiet? It's not much better. Let's look at how to be more trauma-informed.

- **Missed Connection.** Any cue to practice five breaths followed by silence lacks two important opportunities for connection: physical movement connecting mind, body, and breath, and your voice 'as a thread to safety'. Many suggestions on how to teach breathwork to create these key connections are in the next chapter.
- **A Take-home Guide.** Using the same wording can be a helpful guide as someone later may hear your voice in their mind. If you are not saying anything, they have nothing to remember except perhaps the physical unease of wondering if they are doing it right or why you stopped talking. This sensory feeling may be stored as an implicit memory (encoded without words). Therefore, the *feeling* of unease may be what is experienced the next time someone tries to practice any breathwork.
- **Quick Takeaway.** So, do breathwork and talking mix? Yes, but … and it's a big but. The talking needs to be about what you are doing: supporting ways to notice, to feel, and to be curious about the breath.

## Supporting Empowerment

I taught the yoga component in a clinical sexual assault therapy program. I would ask if anyone had done any simple breathwork that week. One woman shared, "I was standing in front of a judge. He stops and says to me, 'Are you okay?' I said, 'Oh yeah, I am just doing my breathing, keep going.'" Another woman shared that her family calls her all the time to make sure she is okay: "So, I am talking to my grandma, and she asks me what's wrong. I was doing our breathing, so I said, 'Nothing's wrong, Gram, just breathe with me now'. So, we did, over the phone." Another shared that she did three minutes of our breathing when she felt a panic attack about to happen in a public place. These women had practiced what Thich Nhat Hanh taught: "Breath is the bridge which connects life to consciousness, which unites your body to your thoughts. Whenever your mind becomes scattered, use your breath as the means to take hold of your mind again" (Hahn, 1975/1999).

**All Together Now – But Not:** A common question is, "How do I match my breath to my clients, patients, or students?" The short answer is you probably cannot, and syncing breaths becomes more improbable with more participants. But more importantly, you should not be trying. A trauma-informed approach empowers someone to find and to practice their own breathing patterns to self-regulate. Your role is as the guide. Your role is not to tell someone how to use their breath.

## What a Difference a Word Makes

We have considered words as potential trauma triggers. Now let's consider how simple word choice can empower someone's breathwork practice. You will find words that resonate with your style, but these ideas provide a solid place from which to start. I have had both clinicians and teachers say, "Oh, I hadn't thought of that – but it makes sense." If your intention is to provide phrases someone can use later or even to share, then think simple, think literal, think non-triggering.

**The Power of YOU:** After the second time an agitated veteran asked me, "Am I breathing right? Is this right?" I realized I had failed. Why was it completely my fault he *felt* unsure? I had externalized his breathing practice: he was responding to me, not connecting with his breath. This realization set me on the path to rework how I taught breathwork based on what I had learned about trauma, the neurobiology of the mind/body connection, and my experiences teaching those with trauma histories. "Breathe in, hands lift," became: "As YOU breathe in, hands lift." What does that slight word change mean to you? I thought including and stressing the word YOU offered three positive points. 1) It builds breath awareness by personalizing the pairing of breathwork and movement. 2) It empowers someone to choose when they want to breathe and to move. 3) Someone who has experienced trauma can feel invisible, not seen and not heard. So, adding the word YOU also acknowledges someone and shows your confidence in their ability to create their own practice today.

**Breathe in or Inhale?** I use the more common phrases breathe in and breathe out, not inhale and exhale. An exception is when teaching Spanish speakers (and there are others), as the words inhale (inhaler) and exhale (exhaler) are similar. 'Simple to understand, Simple to do'.

***Your* Breath or *The* Breath?** Yes, the phrase feel your breath in is simple. But consider that someone who hears your voice later when they need a friendly guide would need to change the wording, which makes it no longer your voice. Set up for success. Feel *the* breath provides ready-to-use consistent phrasing: that is, less work for the verbal part of the brain.

**"Well, you said ..."** Teaching six classes a week to veterans with clinical trauma diagnoses provided many opportunities to iterate my teaching. I wanted words or short phrases to underscore the idea that this class was not yesterday, and that tomorrow might be different. I was already linking breathwork and movement. A simple phrase, "Always breathe in a way that is comfortable for you today," proved a winner. I often had people repeat to me after class, "Well, you said to breathe in a way that is comfortable today." Adding *today* gave a time stamp to what we were doing.

## Of Boundaries and Windows and Personal Growth

**Boundaries:** Cues with a clear end point provide something missing at the time of trauma: boundaries. Verbal boundaries give a framework within which to try new things or to be curious about the process. "If you like, we can practice 5 breaths," or, "The suggestion is to practice 3 breaths as we move in tree pose." Consider what a simple boundary can bring to your program.

- **Consistency.** Your teaching is consistent and predictable because you always specify the number of breaths.
- **Attention.** Someone can focus on their breath. They aren't distracted by such thoughts as: "How long are we doing this? Do I even want to do this, anyway? Shouldn't we be done now?"
- **Window of Tolerance.** It allows people to expand what Daniel Siegel, MD, calls a window of tolerance, which is the time before stress responses kick in (pp. 23–24). A therapist shared with me that a client said, "I usually struggle with my mind wandering and when you said that thing about doing it five times, I was like, I did that. So, that was cool."
- **Keeping Time.** A boundary can be a timekeeper for poses. "The suggestion is to hold the stretch ... but not the breath. Let's practice 2 more breaths here. Feel the breath in ... Feel the breath out." (*Say 2 times*

*slowly.*) People share that this wording helps them feel the breath and the movement. They can *feel* they are not stuck.

- **Personal Growth.** A boundary offers a clear marker from which to assess personal growth. "Today if you like, say the next 2 breaths to yourself in your mind. Take your time with your words … Take your time with your breath."

**Choice:** Many will agree that telling someone to take a few breaths and calm down can elicit the opposite response. A trauma-informed approach is to share nondirective breathwork in ways that encourage curiosity and support making choices, which are again (and again) key steps in trauma recovery and in building resiliency skills (van der Kolk, 2015; Ogden, 2006). "Longer breaths in *can* be energizing. The suggestion is to practice 5 breaths."

## Knowledge Is Power

Presenting one piece of information gives someone the opportunity to make an informed, simple choice. 'Be informed and be inspired' applies to everyone.

**You Had Me at Blood Pressure:** Throughout the practice, in some of the breathwork I will offer one point of information. "Long, slow breaths out *can* lower heart rate, lower blood pressure, and lower muscle tension." Usually, the phrase lowers blood pressure resonates with people. Some veterans were inspired to start a home contest (not my idea) to see who could get their blood pressure down the most with five long, slow breaths out: 35 points was the winner. Thank you, Pocatello telehealth veterans for being inspired.

**Who's in Charge?** One empowering piece of information to share is, "You can manage how you are feeling by managing how you breathe. It's body physiology." I often use the phrase 'It's body physiology' to confirm the ideas are science-based. It celebrates Dr. John Ratey's idea that "… a working knowledge of your brain takes guilt out of the equation." If someone wants more information, I have handouts, or we chat after class (Appendix C: Supplemental Resources).

## Normalize

To normalize means to designate something that happens or a feeling experienced as normal. That is, someone's feelings or differing abilities are not freakish, a personal failure, or a reason to feel guilt or shame. Let's consider some normalizing breathwork strategies.

**Set up for Success:** Someone new to your class or even a regular may find paying attention to the breath today is too many things. "If paying attention to your breath isn't happening for you today, perhaps another day. Always breathe in a comfortable way." At the very least, someone becomes aware paying attention to their breath isn't happening for them today. Sometimes, that gentle permission is all that is needed for someone to reconnect at another time. And of course, it's a good reminder for your group.

**The Pollyanna Approach:** At the end of a practice as you are 'Making a Plan' (p. 211), you could say, "Notice if during this past week you did a 5-part breath. If you did, that's good news. And if you did not, that's good news too. You have a simple, free way to practice changing how you are feeling during the coming week." 'Seeds planted'.

## Maintaining Simplicity

As noted, often those teaching breathwork feel drawn to add extra words or to leave periods of silence. Such teaching styles are not wrong, but they are not trauma-informed.

Be confident there are ways to use 'your voice as a thread to safety' while still keeping it simple.

### Keeping It Simple

Keeping the thread of your voice going brings us back to two key ideas in GreenTREE Yoga® Approach.

**'Trust the Yoga'** As noted several times, Iyengar said that yoga needs to be experienced. And since breathwork is integral to a yoga practice, trust someone can experience the benefits of breathwork without lengthy explanations. A trauma-informed approach begins the yoga practice with breathwork and movement, not with distracting preamble or wordy instructions.

**'Show, Don't Tell'** If you want people to use breathwork to practice self-regulation or to ground or to energize or to reduce stress or to reconnect with bodily sensations, then show specific, real-time ways by pairing simple breathwork to movement. I offer some examples now, with the full scripts in the next chapter. Consider Natalie Babbitt's observation in *Tuck Everlasting* that: "Like all magnificent things, it's very simple."

**Telling:** "You seem stressed, even agitated. Let's do some breathing to help calm down. This really will help you. So, you need to take long breaths out. I know this breathing always makes me feel better."

**Showing:** "Long, slow breaths out *can* lower blood pressure. The suggestion is to practice 5 breaths. On YOUR next breath in, press down on your toes. As YOU breathe out, release."

**Telling:** "You seem tired. There are a lot of different things you can do to feel a bit more energy. This is one of my favorites, it always makes me feel more alert. You really need to take deep breaths in."

**Showing:** "Longer breaths in *can* energize. If you like, let's practice this stretch 3 times. On YOUR longer breath in, arms stretch up. As YOU breathe out, arms release."

**Telling:** "Remember to keep breathing."

**Showing:** "Notice if you are breathing." In a room of yoga teachers, this cue during tree pose often elicits nervous laughter.

**Telling:** "Don't hold your breath."

**Showing:** "When you notice that you are breathing … when you notice you are breathing, wiggle your fingers."

## Literal and Body-based

**Is There Another Route?** A moment of review: Joseph LeDoux, PhD, a renowned neuroscientist, studies the importance of "developing alternate neural pathways to decrease the fear response or anxiety" (LeDoux, 2015). Not pairing simple breathwork with discernable and controllable movements (alternate pathways) seems a lost opportunity to practice another response. The GreenTREE Yoga® Approach pairs simple breathwork with movement, often in the hands or the feet to maximize bodily sensations and awareness. It's a strong tool to empower someone to practice "alternate neural pathways" to the fear response. As the brain rewires over time, this new pathway can become a more adaptive response, perhaps becoming a habit.

**A Soft Purple Light:** What a flowery or more poetic description of the breath lacks, the Stanford neurobiologist Andrew Huberman, PhD, notes, is specificity. Someone has been given nothing "actionable to do in real-time" (Huberman, 2021). Exactly how does the breath moving through every cell of your body feel? Gentle images of breath filling you like a soft purple light may be soothing to some. But to someone in trauma recovery, flowery talk can leave them distracted, trying to figure out what you mean. Body-based cues are both specific and literal, providing a simple way to draw attention to bodily sensations. "Notice if you are breathing in through your nose or in through your mouth. Don't change it, simply notice it."

## Consistent Phrasing

**Why Does Breathwork Begin and End with the Same Cues?** The simple breathwork practices in this book begin with the same cue, "When you are ready, gently press one shoulder back … Then gently press the other shoulder back." The cue signals breathwork is about to happen and that breathwork is worthy of preparation. It also physically prepares someone for more effective breathing by creating more space in the chest and abdomen. Ending with the same cue, "If you like, gently *move* the fingers on one hand or shake that hand … Then gently *move* the fingers on the other hand or shake that hand," provides symmetry to the simple breathwork practice, a grounding opportunity, and a physical stress release.

**Why Repeat?** A clinician shared, "It was a bit shocking and quite humbling. A client told me that during the past week he could hear my voice as he breathes during the week." Consistent breathwork cues can build a stronger program for several reasons. Milton H. Erickson, MD, a renowned psychiatrist and hypnotherapist, entitled one of his books, *My Voice Will Go with You*. The title captures the importance of the human voice as a tool to engage someone in their own healing. In addition to your consistent words as a guide, repetition gives someone more mental energy to notice their breath and bodily sensations. Repetition also can be calming, like a rhythm or a verbal rocking. A therapist shared that he had noticed his resistant clients like the breathwork with five parts because, he thought, the rhythm gave a sense of predictability and control.

**Variations:** Even if the phrases are the same, which they are in the breathing scripts by design, there is still something you can vary. You can vary the prosody of your speech, that is your tone, the emphasis on certain words, and your cadence or pacing. Here is another experiential opportunity. How many ways can you say the word "Goodbye"? It might be amusing to record yourself. Can you say it in a way that conveys being amused, uncertain, curious, forlorn, scared, diffident, rushed, dismissive, distracted, annoyed, sleepy, or disappointed? You can do a lot with your voice with only one word. So you can use the same phrases but vary how you say them. Less for a brain to process but variety to keep the interest. But of course, do not create a distraction with wild swings in intonation or the annoying yoga teacher's voice. 'More is not better, more is confusing.' It's important to remember, you want to sound like yourself. To support your teaching efforts, ideas on how to practice your trauma-informed voice are found in Chapter 5 (p. 110).

## Mixing It up Without Getting Mixed Up

Adding one engaging variation to familiar breathwork can keep your teaching fresh and keep you engaged. People have told me, "I love how you mix it up a bit." There is a balance to be found. As with suggesting options, one variation at a time is a trauma-informed rule of thumb. The next chapter has breathwork scripts with suggested variations to add over time. We will circle back to ways to add variations to the full practice at the end of Chapter 8.

**********

**To Recap:** Breathwork is not an extra part of yoga practice. Yoga is, as Desikachar said, as much a practice involving the breath as it is involving the body. So, considering why breathwork should be a key part of your program is part of teaching preparation for a short break or a full practice. This chapter provides the background to set you up for success as you prepare to practice or to teach the suggested simple breathwork in the next chapter. Trauma-informed breathwork uses strategies key to the GreenTREE Yoga® Approach: building safety, supporting empowerment, and maintaining simplicity.

## References

Desikachar, T.K.V. (1995). *The Heart of Yoga*. Rochester, VT: Inner Traditions International, pp. 18–19; 51.

Erikson, Milton. (1991). *My Voice Will Go with You*. New York: W.W. Norton.

Hahn, Thich Nhat. (1975/1999). *The Miracle of Mindfulness*. Boston: Beacon Press.

Huberman, Andrew. (2021). *Tools for Managing Stress & Anxiety*. Hubermanlab.com. March 8.

Ledoux, Joseph (2015). *Anxious: Using the Brain to Understand and Treat Fear and Anxiety*. New York: Viking, pp. 31–35; 211.

Ogden, Pat. (2006). *Trauma and the Body*. New York. W.W. Norton, pp. 168–169.

Phillips, Dave. (2015). In Unit Stalked by Suicide, Veterans Try to Save One Another. *New York Times*, 9/19.

Porges, Stephe. (2011). *The Pocket Guide to the Polyvagal Theory: The Transformative Power of Feeling Safe*. New York: W.W. Norton, p. 109.

Van der Kolk, Bessel. (2015). *The Body Keeps the Score: Brain, Mind, and Body in the Healing of Trauma*. New York: Penguin Publishing, pp. 208–209.

# 7
# Suggested Breathwork

## At the Ready: Ways to Ground throughout the Practice

As you read the breathwork scripts, notice the simple cues that support making choices and building body awareness. It's always worth another mention that linking simple breathwork to the many sense receptors in the hands and feet supports a feeling of grounding (being in the present). The following 'Show, Don't Tell' ideas can be used to start a practice or between flows during the practice. Grounding techniques can also be effective to start, to end, or to turn any clinical or health care session around. Downloads of MP3s and MP4s of some breathwork and practice scripts are available to support your personal and professional efforts to build resiliency skills and to support trauma recovery (Appendix C: Supplemental Resources).

1. **'The Shifting Breath'** (photo p. 242) (standing or seated)

   1) "When you are ready, gently press one shoulder back ... Then press the other shoulder back. The suggestion is to practice 3 'Shifting Breaths' with your palms facing forward. As YOU breathe in, shift forward. ... As YOU breathe out, release. (*Say 3 times slowly.*)
   2) Now let's practice 3 'Shifting Breaths' with palms facing back. Keeping a gentle bend in your knees can protect your knee joints.

   As YOU breathe in, shift back ... As YOU breathe out, release. (*Say 3 times slowly.*)

   3) If you like, gently *stretch* the fingers on one hand or shake that hand ... Then gently *stretch* the fingers on the other hand or shake that hand. Let your hands be as still as you would like them to be."

   **Variation:** "As YOU breathe in, palms forward, shift forward, today your *heels* may lift ... As YOU breathe out, release. Notice if you have a slight

DOI: 10.4324/9781003308836-10

bend in your knees. On YOUR next breath in, palms back, shift back, *toes* lift ... As YOU breathe out, release." (*Say 3 times slowly.*)

2. **Hands, Feet, Fingers, and Toes**

   a. **Standing: Hands on Hips**

      1) "When you are ready, gently press one shoulder back ... Then press the other shoulder back.
      2) If you like, put your hands on your hips. The suggestion is to practice 3 breaths.

      As YOU breathe in, press down on your hands ... As YOU breathe out, release the press. (*Say 3 times slowly.*)

      3) If you like, gently *stretch* the fingers on one hand or shake that hand ... Then gently *stretch* the fingers on the other hand or shake that hand."

   b. **Seated: Pressing Hands or Fingertips**

      1) "When you are ready, gently press one shoulder back ... Then press the other shoulder back.
      2) If you like, put your hands on the sides of your chair (or fingertips on the floor). The suggestion is to practice 3 breaths. As YOU breathe in, press down on your hands ... As YOU breathe out, release the press. (*Say 3 times slowly.*)
      3) When you are ready, gently *stretch* the fingers on one hand or shake that hand ... Then gently *stretch* the fingers on the other hand or shake that hand."

   c. **Seated: Hands on Legs:** I was surprised at the number of positive comments when I first taught this simple breath.

      1) "When you are ready, gently press one shoulder back ... Then press the other shoulder back.
      2) If you like, put your hands on your legs. The suggestion is to practice 3 breaths.
      3) As YOU breathe in, press down on your hands ... As YOU breathe out, release the press. (*Say 3 times slowly.*)

4) If you like, gently *wiggle* the fingers on one hand or shake that hand … Then gently *wiggle* the fingers on the other hand or shake that hand."

d. **Seated or Standing: Toes**

1) "When you are ready, gently press one shoulder back … Then press the other shoulder back.
2) The suggestion is to practice 3 breaths. As YOU breathe in, toes press … As YOU breathe out, release. (*Say 3 times slowly.*)
3) If you like, gently *stretch* your toes on one foot or shake that foot. Then gently *stretch* your toes on the other foot or shake that foot."

e) **Mix and Match – Hands and Feet:** Use this variation after everyone is familiar with these breaths.

1) "If you like, put your hands on your hips. The suggestion is to practice 5 breaths.

As YOU breathe in, press down on one *hand* … As YOU breathe out, release.

As YOU breathe in, press down on the *other hand* … As YOU breathe out, release.

As YOU breathe in, press down on one *foot* … As YOU breathe out, release.

As YOU breathe in, press down on the *other foot* … As YOU breathe out, release.

As YOU breathe in, you choose, press down on *one hand* and *one foot*."

(**Or:** *opposite* hand and foot **or** *both* hands and both feet.)

**Variations:**

1) **Texture:** "Notice the texture under your hands (fingertips or toes)." **Or:** 2) **Vary the Press:** Vary the press for each cue: either firm or gentle. "As YOU breathe in, press (firmly/gently) on your toes … As YOU breathe out, release." **Or:** 3) **Notice the Press:** If your cue is simply to press down on your hands, at the end say, "Notice if you pressed gently or firmly. Simply notice."

### 3. Go Big

We usually don't think of large movements as grounding. But large movements done in rhythm with the breath can reduce general anxiety and give visceral cues of being present.

#### a. 'Arms Stretch/Hands Press'

1) "If you like, we can practice the 'Arms Stretch/Hands Press' 3 times. Always breathe and move in a way that is comfortable today.

As YOU breathe in, look up, stretch up, *palms* press overhead …

As YOU breathe out, arms release, palms tap legs. (*Say 3 times slowly.*)

If you like, gently *stretch* the fingers on one hand or shake that hand … Then gently *stretch* the fingers on the other hand or shake that hand."

**Variation:** "As YOU breathe in, look up, stretch up, *fingertips* press overhead … As YOU breathe out, *fingertips* tap legs."

#### b. 'Arms Stretch/Toes Press'

1) "If you like, we can practice 'Arms Stretch/Toes Press' 3 times. Always move in a way that is comfortable for you today. As YOU breathe in, look up, *stretch* up, toes press …

As YOU breathe out, arms release, toes release.
(*Say slowly 2 more times.*)

2) If you like, gently *stretch* your toes on one foot or shake that foot. Then gently *stretch* your toes on the other foot or shake the other foot."

## Five-breath Format

### Opening Comments

**Format:** Getting set up to do breathwork is part of empowering someone to self-regulate. As you might expect, the setup involves movement. Ten breathwork practices with variations use this format: setup/five-part breath/ending. The same format provides an empowering base of familiarity, consistency, and learning through repetition. It also simplifies your teaching. And, again, should someone want to practice later, your supportive words may go with them. Variations engage interest and curiosity without changing the predictable flow.

**The Facts of Breath**

1) **Breath facts** are included in some of the breathwork. "Longer breaths in *can* be energizing," or "Longer breaths out *can* lower blood pressure and lower heart rate." You can select the fact based on your teaching intentions for that part of the practice. Again, the cue uses the word *can* instead of *will* because for some either breathing pattern can be agitating.

2) **Placing the breath fact** you choose between two movement cues prevents talking *at* someone without a physical action to do. The suggested placement is between pressing the shoulders back and putting one or both hands over the heart. The place for your choice is indicated in the script by: (*Your choice of breath fact to share.*)

3) **Adding a breath fact** sometimes can be distracting.

For example, the breathwork in Ways to Ground, the last four breaths of the Five-Breath Format, and Other Breathwork Ideas have enough to consider. For someone fatigued from sleep or pain issues, 'More is not better, more is confusing'. You decide if a breath fact adds to the experience or confuses it. And what is it called if someone practices long breaths in (or out) without your breath fact cue? It is called breath management in action.

**Eyes Open, Eyes Closed:** "Eyes open or eyes closed, your choice. I keep my eyes open so I can let you know if someone joins us," offers an option. "When you are ready, open your eyes," provides the ending. When I don't include these cues, a comment I hear is: "Wow, I closed my eyes, which surprised me." You decide when the eyes open or eyes closed, your choice cue can be useful.

## Ten Breathwork Ideas

1. **'Feel the Breath':** Including 'Feel the Breath' in every practice sets someone up for success. I find it is the simplest breath to do and to remember, which is why I teach it in all practices. As I mentioned, cuing *the* breath and not *your* breath means no words changes if someone hears your voice later. In all things: simple, simple, simple. The suggestion is to introduce any variations slowly over several practices. Yet including the most basic 'Feel the Breath' first in every practice sets the scene and provides consistency.

   1) "When you are ready, gently press one shoulder back … Then press the other shoulder back.
   2) (*Your choice of breath fact to share.*)
   3) "If you like, put one or both hands over your heart … Put one or both hands over your heart.

4) The suggestion is to practice 'Feel the Breath' 5 times. Feel the breath in … Feel the breath out. (*Say 2 times slowly.*) Always breathe in a comfortable way. Feel the breath in … Feel the breath out. (*Say 3 times slowly.*)

5) If you like, gently *move* the fingers on one hand or shake that hand … Then gently *move* the fingers on the other hand or shake that hand."

**Variations:** Make the following changes to 'Feel the Breath'.

**Variation 1: 'Finger Press Breath':** Change # 4): "The suggestion is to practice 'Finger Press Breath' 5 times. Feel the breath in, fingers press … Feel the breath out, release the press. (*Say 2 times slowly.*) Always breathe in a comfortable way. Feel the breath in, fingers press … Feel the breath out, release the press." (*Say 3 times slowly.*)

**Variation 2: Choose a Breathing Pattern:** Change #2): "Based on how you are feeling right now, choose a breathing pattern. Longer breaths in *can* be energizing. Longer breaths out *can* lower heart rate, lower blood pressure, and lower muscle tension." Change # 4): "The suggestion is to practice five breaths using the breathing pattern you choose today."

**Variation 3a: 'You Are Always with You':** A veteran shared with me, and others agreed, that the phrase 'because you are always with you' had such a positive impact on her. It told her she was enough, that she could take care of herself.

Add to #4): After 2 (or 3) breaths, (depending on the group) "Now if you like, because you are always with you, say the next 2 (or 3) breaths to yourself in your mind … say the next 2 (or 3) breaths to yourself in your mind". The idea is not to leave dead air and to keep 'your voice as a thread to safety'. Say slowly with pauses to fill the length of 3 breaths: "Don't rush your breath … Don't rush your words … Take your time with your breath … Take your time with your words."

**Variation 3b: Notice If You Said All Three Breaths to Yourself:** Can you *feel* why the following cues could be perceived as a negative while distracting from the task at hand, which is noticing the breath? "Notice where your mind wandered," could set off a chain of thoughts and *feelings* unrelated to the breath. To put a finer point on this idea, that simple cue could lead to: "Oh, well, I started thinking about that time when …" The cue: "Notice if you weren't able to pay attention," could make someone feel, well, as though they failed at another simple thing. A clinician told me a client shared, "I was only able to get to three breaths before I lost concentration. Different days, different attention." The client used a variation on what the clinician had said in session: "Different days, different stretches." To maintain focus on the breath, "Notice where your mind wandered," can become: "Notice if you said all three breaths to yourself. Simply notice. Either way, it's good news. If you did, you have a tool ready to use. If you didn't, it's still good news. You have a quick, easy, free way to manage your stress ready to practice this week."

2. **'Fist Breathing' ('Open and Close Breath'):** Working with veterans, I was looking for a new name for fist breathing. But a fourth grader told me, "I felt like putting my fist through a wall, so I did fist breathing instead." I checked with my veterans' groups and decided to keep what seemed a positive repurposing of the word fist. This name has worked with my groups. However, an astute teacher made an adjustment. In her refugee class, one woman with a black eye braced at the use of the word fist. 'Fist Breathing' became 'Open and Close Breath'. A clinician told me she called it 'Rock and Flower Breath' with children. Choose names that meet your trauma-informed teaching intentions.

You may work with people who have fibromyalgia, arthritis, or finger/hand pain from injury, torture, or abuse. Someone having a low-energy day may be doing the practice lying down as you suggested, "breathing and moving in ways that feel comfortable to you today." One day I observed someone with gnarled, arthritic fingers and someone with painful fibromyalgia. Wanting to set them up for success, I found an inclusive way to build more body awareness into the breathwork for everyone.

1) "When you are ready, gently press one shoulder back ... Then press the other shoulder back.

2) The suggestion is to try one or more of these four ways to move your fingers with me now. (*Say slowly as you do each one together to keep everyone engaged.*) The first is moving your fingers a small amount. Another way is pressing four fingers on your thumbs. Or today you might gently press your fingers on your palms. The last suggestion is to make tight fists, maybe so tight you feel your forearms and face tighten.

3) (*Your choice of breath fact to share.*)

4) If you like, choose one way to move your fingers as we practice 'Fist Breathing' ('Open and Close Breath') 5 times.

As YOU breathe in, fingers move ... As YOU breathe out, release. (*Say 2 times slowly.*)

Always breathe and move in a comfortable way.

On YOUR next breath in, fingers move ... As YOU breathe out, release.

As YOU breathe in, fingers move ... As YOU breathe out, release. (*Repeat last cue slowly.*)

5) If you like, gently *wiggle* the fingers on one hand or shake that hand ... Then gently *wiggle* the fingers on the other hand or shake that hand."

**Variation:** To extend opportunities for both body awareness and choice offer: "Today you may like to try moving your fingers in a *new* way, one you haven't done before." Did you notice that even doing it the same way is still a choice? But someone may expand their window of tolerance by being curious and trying something new in the safety of your trauma-informed space.

3. **'The Finger Stretch Breath':**

1) "When you are ready, gently press one shoulder back ... Then press the other shoulder back.
2) (*Your choice of breath fact to share.*)
3) The suggestion is to practice 'The Finger Stretch Breath' 5 times.

   As YOU breathe in, fingers stretch ... As YOU breathe out, release the stretch. (*Say 2 times slowly.*)  Always breathe and move in a comfortable way.

   On YOUR next breath in, fingers stretch ... As YOU breathe out, release the stretch.

   As YOU breathe in, fingers stretch ... As YOU breathe out, release the stretch. (*Say 2 times slowly.*)

4) If you like, gently *close* the fingers on one hand or shake that hand ... Then gently *close* the fingers on the other hand or shake that hand."

**Variation: 'Finger Flow':** "Let's practice 'Finger Flow' 3 times on one hand and then the 3 times on the other hand. As YOU breathe in, fingers open ... As YOU breathe out, move one finger at a time toward your palm." (Breath 2 and 3: "As YOU breathe out, fingers flow."
(*Say 3 times slowly. Repeat on other side.*)

**More variations:** 1) Practice starting with the forefinger on one hand and the little finger on the other; **Or:** 2) Don't specify and at the end ask someone to notice how they flowed; **Or:** 3) Suggest someone choose how to move their fingers *today*.

### 4. 'Fingertip Breathing':

This breathwork creates a gentle rhythm of breath and movement guided by the many sense receptors in the fingertips and palms.

1) "When you are ready, gently press one shoulder back … Then press the other shoulder back.
2) (Your choice of breath fact to share.)
3) Put your hands together as if they are around a ball. Perhaps today it is comfortable to rest your hands in your lap.
4) If you like, press your fingertips firmly together. Then change the press to a gentle one, perhaps fingertips barely touching.
5) The suggestion is to practice 'Fingertip Breathing' 5 times.

As YOU breathe in, firm press … As YOU breathe out, gentle press. (*Say 2 times slowly.*)

Always move and breathe in a comfortable way.

On YOUR next breath in, firm press … As YOU breathe out, gentle press.

As YOU breathe in, firm press … As YOU breathe out, gentle press. (*Repeat last cue slowly.*)

6) If you like, gently *stretch* the fingers on one hand or shake that hand … Then gently *stretch* the fingers on the other hand or shake that hand."

**Variation: 'Palm Press' ('Balloon Breath'):** Fingertips remain pressing together for both the breaths in and breaths out. "As YOU breathe in, palms apart … As YOU breathe out, palms press." (*Say 5 times slowly.*) This breath is fun to name as a group.

### 5. 'The Wave Breath': (photo on p. 242 (c) and (d))

You are doing the breathwork too, so you do not have to verbally cue hand movements. If you are seated, palms turn up on the breath in and turn down on the breath out. The shared ideas for renaming this breath are creative, fun, and build social connection. Some veterans named this 'The Wave Breath'.

1) "When you are ready, gently press one shoulder back … Then press the other shoulder back.
2) (Your choice of breath fact to share.)
3) The suggestion is to practice 'The Wave Breath' 5 times.

As YOU breathe in, hands lift (*palms up*) … As YOU breathe out, release (*palms down*). (*Say 2 times slowly.*) Always breathe in a comfortable way. On YOUR next breath in, hands lift … As YOU breathe out, release. As YOU breathe in, hands lift … As YOU breathe out, release. (*Repeat last cue slowly.*)

4) If you like, gently *stretch* the fingers on one hand or shake that hand … Then gently *stretch* the fingers on the other hand or shake that hand."

## 6. The 'Anytime, Anywhere Breath':

Some women shared that talk therapy could be triggering. We came up with an idea that proved quite helpful. I teach this breath to all groups around the holidays.

1) "You can do the 'Anytime, Anywhere Breath' seated or standing, eyes open or eyes closed, in a group, even when you are talking with someone.
2) When you are ready, gently press one shoulder back … Then press the other shoulder back. If you like, place one hand on your leg.
3) The suggestion is to practice long, slow breaths out if that is comfortable today.
4) Let's practice 5 breaths. As YOU breathe in, fingers press … As YOU breathe out, release. (*Say 2 times slowly.*) Always breathe in a comfortable way. On YOUR next breath in, fingers press … As YOU breathe out, release. As YOU breathe in, fingers press … As YOU breathe out, release. (*Repeat last cue slowly.*)
5) When you are ready, gently *move* the fingers on one hand or shake that hand … Then gently *move* the fingers on the other hand or shake that hand."

**Variations:** 1) "Press your fingers firmly (or gently) today." **Or:** 2) "Now if you like, use your other hand and practice saying it 3 times to yourself in your mind, since *you* are always with you." Say slowly during this time so you don't leave dead air: "Don't rush your words … Don't rush your breath … Take your time with your words … Take your time with your breath."

## 7. The ATM Breath:

Moshe Feldenkrais, PhD, brilliant as both a physicist and somatically based healer, created a program called Awareness Through Movement (ATM). He believed that smaller movements created better body awareness. Dr. Feldenkrais taught that the more subtle the movement, the more awareness you can build (Feldenkrais, 1972). An interesting side note: in 1939, Dr. Feldenkrais worked in the lab of the Nobel Prize winners, the Curies, developing the particle accelerator that split the uranium atom. Later, through his foundational body work programs, he proved to be one of the first neuroplasticians (Doidge, 2015).

1) "When you are ready, gently press one shoulder back … Then press the other shoulder back. (*No breathing pattern cue so full attention can be on the small movements of this breathwork.*)
2) If you like, let's practice 5 breaths, moving your fingers simply enough to notice the movement.
3) As YOU breathe in, fingers move enough to notice … As YOU breathe out, fingers release. (*Say 2 times slowly.*) Always breathe and move in a comfortable way.

On YOUR next breath in, fingers move … As YOU breathe out, fingers release.

As YOU breathe in, fingers move enough to notice … As YOU breathe out, fingers release. (*Repeat last cue slowly.*)

4) If you like, gently *move* the fingers on one hand or shake that hand … Then gently *move* the fingers on the other hand or shake that hand."

8. **Notice What Moves as You Breathe:**

I've been told these cues bring awareness to someone holding their breath. (*No breathing pattern cue cue so full attention on the small movements of this breathwork.*)

1) "When you are ready, gently press one shoulder back … Then press the other shoulder back.
2) If you like, put one or both hands over your heart … Put one or both hands over your heart.
3) The suggestion is to practice 5 breaths. As YOU breathe in, notice what moves … As YOU breathe out, notice what moves. (*Say 2 times slowly.*) Always breathe in a comfortable way. Next time YOU breathe in, notice what moves … As YOU breathe out, notice what moves.

As YOU breathe in, notice what moves … As YOU breathe out, notice what moves.

(*Repeat last cue slowly.*)

4) If you like, gently *move* the fingers on one hand or shake that hand, then gently *move* the fingers on the other hand or shake that hand."

9.  **'Goal Post Breathing' with 'It's a Wrap': (a./b.)** (photo on p. 141 (a)–(c))

This breath was inspired by breathwork Bessel van der Kolk taught at four workshops I attended. I added the fingertip press to access the dense sensory pathways and allow for fingertip variations. A complementary breath is 'It's a Wrap' to experience being in control of containment after being in control of openness. This sequence was contributed by Elizabeth Q. Finlinson, LCSW.

a.  **'Goal Post Breathing':**

1) "When you are ready, gently press one shoulder back … Then press the other shoulder back. (*No breathing pattern cue as the nature of the movement will lengthen each breath.*)

2) The suggestion is to practice 'Goal Post Breathing' 5 times. With each breath in, you can move your hands farther apart, in any way that is comfortable today.

As YOU breathe in, hands apart … As YOU breathe out, fingertips press. As YOU breathe in, hands a little farther apart … As YOU breathe out, fingertips press.

Always breathe and move in a comfortable way.

On YOUR next breath in, hands a little farther apart … As YOU breathe out, fingertips press. As YOU breathe in, hands a little farther apart … As YOU breathe out, fingertips press." (*Repeat last cue slowly.*)

**Variations:** 1) Specify a firm fingertip press or a light fingertip press each time; **Or:** 2) Cue the first 2 as firm and the last 3 as gentle; **Or:** 3) Cue the first with firm press, the second with gentle press, and the last 3 cues with no suggestions. At the end, "Notice the press you chose to do for the last 3 breaths."

b.  **'It's a Wrap':** The simple act of wrapping arms around oneself can ground. Perhaps refrain from mentioning the benefits of giving yourself a well-earned hug because you are important. Again, not wrong. But such musings are distracting and could be triggering. "Have I earned a hug?" Or "Do I care about myself, no one else seems to." Or "I don't like to be hugged," and well, you get the idea. I do not even use the word hug or squeeze. Using a less reactive word supports focusing on body-based sensations. Visual cues reduce the need for extra verbal cues to process.

1) "Now if you like, create a comfortable arm wrap. (*No breathing pattern cue.*)

2) The suggestion is to practice 3 breaths in 'It's a Wrap'. As YOU breathe in, fingers gently press ... As YOU breathe out, release the press. (*Say 3 times slowly.*)

3) If you like, create a wrap with the other arm on top. (*Repeat.*)

4) When you are ready, gently *move* the fingers on one hand or shake that hand ... Then gently *move* the fingers on the other hand or shake that hand."

**Variations:** 1) "The suggestion is to take longer breaths in and notice how it feels." You may want to try it first, as it creates an interesting breath sensation as you literally breathe into the stretch. People share that they like the interesting feeling. However, consider the following. From my work with autism, I thought a helpful cue would be to press on the arms too. I am grateful to a talented yoga teacher who reminded me that constrained feeling as a cue could be triggering. Thank you, Rebecca! Lesson learned: we always need to be learning. **Or:** 2) Guide varying finger movements with one simple choice: "If you like, tap your fingers." Or "If you like, find your own rhythm, perhaps strumming." Or "If you like, tap slowly or quickly".

## 10. 'Stop Sign Breath' (photo on p. 241 (d) and (e))

These hand motions allow for completing the action of pushing something away, something that may have been denied at the time of trauma. For the full story on how this breath came to be (p. 137).

1) "When you are ready, gently press one shoulder back ... Then press the other shoulder back.

2) (*No breathing pattern cue.*) The suggestion is to practice the 'Stop Sign Breath' 5 times.

As YOU breathe in, palms press forward, (ONLY *you softly say 'stop'*) ... As YOU breathe out, fingers down. (*Say 2 times slowly.*)

Always move and breathe in a comfortable way.

On YOUR next breath in, palms press forward, (*stop*) ... As YOU breathe out, fingers down.

As YOU breathe in, palms forward, (*stop*) ... As YOU breathe out, fingers down. (*Repeat last cue slowly.*)

3) If you like, gently *wiggle* the finger on one hand or shake that hand, then gently *wiggle* the fingers on the other hand or shake that hand."

## Other Breathwork Ideas

Again, there are no breathing pattern cues offered in this breathwork to support full attention to breathing sensations and movement. Keep it simple. Again, someone may choose a breathing pattern without your suggestion, which is breath management in action. Adapt as meets your personal and professional needs.

1. **Thumb to Fingertips Breathing:** Someone told me she couldn't feel her hands until we did this breathing at the end of 'Final Stretch'.

   1) "When you are ready, gently press one shoulder back (or down) ... Then press the other shoulder back (or down). We always do both sides, one hand at a time.
   2) As YOU breathe in, *forefinger* to thumb, gentle press ... As YOU breathe out, release.

   As YOU breathe in, *middle* finger to thumb, gentle press ... As YOU breathe out, release.

   As YOU breathe in, *ring* finger to thumb, gentle press ... As YOU breathe out, release.

   As YOU breathe in, *little* finger to thumb, gentle press ... As YOU breathe out, release.

   3) Now let's use the other hand with a firm press if you like. Always breathe in a comfortable way. **(Repeat using a firm press cue on the other hand.)**
   4) If you like, gently *move* the fingers on one hand or shake that hand ... Then gently *move* the fingers on the other hand or shake that hand."

2. **More Noticing Breaths**

   a. **Notice Your Breathing:** The breath offers a simple idea and then allows someone to choose.

      1) "When you are ready, gently press one shoulder back ... Then press the other shoulder back.
      2) The suggestion is to practice 2 breaths. Feel the breath in ... Feel the breath out. (*Say 2 times slowly.*) Notice if you breathed in through your mouth or in through your nose. If you like, practice 2 more breaths and change how you are breathing in some way. Feel the breath in ... Feel the breath out." (*Say 2 times slowly.*)

b. **Notice the Pause Breath:** The simple idea of pausing and then noticing the pause is offered, one that supports choice and breath awareness.

   1) "When you are ready, gently press one shoulder back … Then press the other shoulder back.
   2) Let's practice 3 breaths. Today you may like to put a pause between the breath in and the breath out.
   3) As YOU are ready, breathe in … pause so that you notice the pause … Then breathe out. (*Say 3 times slowly.*)
   4) If you like, gently *move* the fingers on one hand or shake that hand, then gently *move* the fingers on the other hand or shake that hand."

**Variations:** 1) "The suggestion is to practice 2 more breaths putting a pause between the breath out and the next breath in." **Or:** 2) "The suggestion is to practice two more breaths and simply notice if you pause as you breathe."

**********

**To Recap:** Breathwork is a key part of any yoga practice, so how you *teach* breathwork is a key part of any yoga practice. Considering yourself as a guide, not a guru, is a way to build a sense of safety and to empower someone to find the breathwork that helps them build simple and effective self-regulation and resiliency skills. This chapter presents some easy-to-use and easy-to-remember breathwork scripts with background information on some breaths in the hopes of inspiring your program. Some downloadable MP3s, MP4s, and practice scripts are available to support your personal and professional efforts to build resiliency skills and support trauma recovery (Appendix C: Supplemental Resources).

## References

Feldenkrais, Moshe. (1972). *Awareness Through Movement*. New York: Harper One.

Doidge, Norman. (2015). *The Brain's Way of Healing: Remarkable Discoveries and Recoveries from the Frontiers of Neuroplasticity*. New York: Penguin Life, p. 169

# 8
# The Practice
## Considerations

---

Teaching the physical practice creates the synergistic interplay between breath and movement and is strengthened by three key trauma-informed ideas: building safety, supporting empowerment, and maintaining simplicity. It is time well spent to review why these three considerations, first discussed in the chapters on language and the breath, are important to planning and then to teaching the yoga practice. Bessel van der Kolk wrote that, "Only by getting in touch with your body, by connecting viscerally with yourself, can you regain a sense of who you are ... you need to get back in touch with your body, with your Self" (van der Kolk, 2015).

I presented at an Institute on Violence, Abuse, and Trauma (IVAT) conference at which a Lakota woman and her granddaughter spoke about the high rates of teen suicide. Later, I asked the granddaughter what they are offering their youth. They are going back to what they know: sweat lodges, group dancing, and burning sage. Many cultures have long used body-based, rhythmic activities that support activating the social engagement system to heal trauma.

Many experts would agree that the benefits of talk therapy are better realized when someone feels safe in their body. Instead of ignoring the body or making it lie still, let's consider why the trauma-informed physical practice (the poses or asana) can be a key part of your teaching, your clinical practice, or your personal recovery plan. This chapter discusses the importance of *why* somatic resourcing needs to be part of trauma recovery, as stressed in the works of Pat Ogden, PhD; Peter Levine, PhD; Gabor Maté, MD; and Bessel van der Kolk, MD. The following chapter discusses *how* to create your practice.

DOI: 10.4324/9781003308836-11

## Building Safety

We have discussed why arranging the yoga space and managing the people in that space play key roles in building a sense of safety. Now let's consider why bringing this same awareness to planning and to teaching is so important.

## Self-regulation

It can be instructive to tease apart Bessel van der Kolk's simple statement: "Self-regulation depends on having a friendly relationship with your body" (van der Kolk, 2015). *Self-regulation* means someone manages their nervous system. The word *friendly* recognizes the reciprocity in the relationship. In other words, the mind is not trying to dominate or to ignore the body. Finally, the phrase *your body* recognizes that to respond in an adaptive way to stressors, someone needs first to notice themselves. They need to notice their physical and emotional sensations.

**Get Moving:** The longer answer to why movement is important for self-regulation is at the end of Chapter 1. The shorter answer is that for many years experts in the field of body-based healing modalities, Moshe Feldenkrais, Fredreick Alexander, Pat Ogden, Peter Levine, Daniel Siegel, and Bessel van der Kolk to name but a few, have advocated using the body as a tool to calm, to heal, and to reset the nervous system.

Again, Pat Ogden and others in the trauma field echo Pierre Janet's from 1925: the positive effect of physically working through an action that was impossible at the time of trauma (Ogden, 2006). As she says, "We need movement to change procedural memory." Procedural (implicit) memory is encoded without words. These memories, including some traumatic ones, are stored in areas of the brain below conscious awareness. Moving also can release muscle stress. After reading her book, *Trauma and the Body*, I began to work subtle body gestures into my teaching. A woman came to my class following military sexual trauma group therapy. As we went around the circle sharing what we noticed about the practice, she shared, and because I wrote it down, I quote, "When we did the breathing with the hands (and she kept repeating the stop gesture as she spoke), I felt like I was pushing at all the negative forces in my life. Just stopping it, pushing it away." Thank you, Pat Ogden (see 'Stop Sign Breath', pp. 199–200).

**Get Organized:** As noted and worth repeating, one of my favorite ideas from Bessel van der Kolk is: "In some ways, yoga organizes your attentional system into very specific movements and postures and keeps you away from the free-floating residue that comes up when you do meditation" (NICABM, #2). Building a physical feeling and a rhythm of flow can organize the attentional system. It can allow someone on a visceral (subcortical) level to experience the feeling they are not stuck. Things are moving. The breath is moving, the body is moving, the breath and body are moving together. Perhaps the group is breathing and moving together as well. That rhythm and connection to both oneself and to others is one way to activate the social engagement system.

As I was teaching warrior two flows to veterans with clinical PTSD diagnoses and varying levels of fitness, it occurred to me that I had a wonderful opportunity to practice flowing with the breath. That is, I could teach large body movements clearly linked to simple breathwork. Why would I want to do this? We know movement can reduce stress, so consider the increased benefits of using the breath to organize large movements in a group. Some teachers mention the breath, yet some can teach an hour with barely a reference. A lost opportunity. As I taught this consistent pairing of simple breathwork and movement in my workshops and trainings, I noticed that many comments from participants included, "I loved how we really moved with the breath, how we flowed." Of note is that I had never mentioned my reasons for teaching in this way. 'Show, Don't Tell'.

## Pacing

Consider the body-based activity of eating. The pace at which we eat affects our digestive, circulatory, muscular, respiratory, and nervous systems. There is also a physiological effect when we talk, move, or breathe quickly. Let's review why the pace at which you teach (speaking and moving) is a tool in body-based modality of trauma-informed yoga. Many find pacing one of the more challenging parts of trauma-informed teaching.

**The Gift of Time:** If your intention is to empower someone, then a question is, "Am I allowing enough time for someone to process my simple suggestion? Am I then allowing enough time for someone to do what I have suggested 'in a way that feels comfortable to you today'?" As a therapist told me, "Always a good reminder to slow down and give time to process and to practice."

**Too Much of a Good Thing:** Some teachers hold a pose for the length of time it takes to finish telling a story or for the most fit person to fall out of the pose. While these approaches may provide some benefit at some time to someone, neither is trauma-informed. While holding a pose can allow time for processing and noticing, putting a boundary on the length of time makes it trauma-informed. Someone knows what to expect. "The suggestion is to practice 3 breaths as we move in warrior two. As YOU breathe in arms lift, fingers stretch wide … as YOU breathe out, release." (*Say 3 times slowly.*)

**Not Enough of a Good Thing:** Quickly moving from pose to pose can take away the opportunity to explore suggestions. Your suggestion is only the first part. Again, the second is giving someone time to process the suggestion. If our intention is to build awareness, then we should teach in a way that supports Moshe Feldenkrais's observation that: "The delay between thought and action is the basis for awareness" (Feldenkrais, 1972/1977). The third part, then, is observing how that action *feels*.

**What's the Rush?** Several concerns can cause you to go too fast. Your focus may be on what is next. Or you rush because you planned too much, or you are nervous. You might think people will be bored. Two simple fixes: practicing your trauma-informed phrasing and planning your classes carefully, both covered in the next chapter.

## 'Your Voice Is a Thread to Safety'

While it is true that other people can cause trauma, it is also true that other people can be instrumental in trauma recovery and in building resiliency skills. Be confident that how you sound and your facial expressions are highly effective tools to use (or misuse). Let's consider your voice.

**More Than Just a Voice:** I remember years ago when I first heard a yoga teacher say their goal was to teach without actually doing the poses. Having spent many years teaching preschoolers to college sciences, I remember thinking that was not a helpful approach. Humans with sight are visual learners, and any group can contain diverse learning styles. Years later, as I studied the neuroscience of safety and of learning, I came to more fully appreciate the reasons for my initial reaction.

Teaching with such verbal clarity that someone does not need to look at you is a fine goal. However, consider that relying on verbal cues alone to a sighted group can limit your effectiveness. Another consideration is that if you are only talking, the perception could be you are watching, judging, and looking for ways to correct.

**Limited Edition:** Why does offering only verbal instructions limit someone's options for processing information? There is no option to listen at times or to look at times or to do a bit of both. There is no option to experience one modality supporting the other. If 'different days, different stretches' is true, so too is 'different days, different modalities'. Someone may be attending to your visual cues as they attune to the rhythms of your breath and movement. A visual cue can also simplify understanding. Someone then can shift attention to noticing their breath, to how a pose *feels*, and to trying something new.

A self-aware person told me she had started doing yoga and always kept her eyes closed. After two years, she started to practice with her eyes open, a personal sign, she said, "of healing from some deep traumas." Perhaps a way to refine a teaching goal would be to teach with such verbal clarity that someone does not have to look at you but also to teach in a way that offers visual cues. 'Simple to understand. Simple to do'.

**Be a Model – No, Not That Kind …** Another reason to do the yoga as you teach is it keeps you engaged. If you are bored, you probably sound bored. Another plus is it can guide some teaching ideas. As I felt my leg muscles working in warrior two, I was inspired to say, "When you feel the muscles in your front leg working … when you feel the muscles in your front leg working, wiggle your fingers." This simple, body-based cue proved so popular I use some variation in every class.

Some yoga studios have mirrors, but let's consider another mirror. The neuroscientist Giacomo Rizzolatti first identified mirroring neurons in monkeys in the 1980s (Rizzolatti, 2004). Research and discovery are ongoing, but as we observe someone, certain brain activities mirror their actions or feelings. You may have experienced how your mood can change by watching others. Such phrases as 'she's the life of the party' or 'he's a wet blanket' come to mind.

How does the science in Chapter 1 underscore the importance of practicing the yoga as we teach? As you teach, changes in your physiological state are embodied in the tone, rhythm, and modulation of your voice. These changes happen as the muscles in the throat and larynx and the muscles of your face respond to signals of stress and safety. You may move through a challenging pose to a point in which breathwork and movement have lowered your stress levels. You have demonstrated the yoga principle of balancing effort (*sthira*) and ease (*sukah*). As someone watches or listens, they can notice or sense that you are not stuck. You have self-regulated. 'It's body physiology' is yet another compelling reason to practice the yoga and not just talk about it.

## Adjustments

Ah, to adjust or not to adjust? Why is that a question, and a good one at that? A few considerations clarify the answer. Some may feel they have not gotten their money's worth if a teacher doesn't adjust their poses. Certainly, one should not say that hands-on adjustments are wrong. But one can say touching students or clients in a yoga class is not trauma-informed. While the healing power of human touch is a tool some use well, it is not within the scope of this book to address when and how to use touch to heal.

**Of Talent and Personal Space:** I will note the teachers in these examples are extremely talented and committed to teaching and studying yoga. Once in downward dog, one teacher lay over me from behind, put her hands on my inner thighs, and outwardly rotated them. I had no idea she was going to do that. She was quietly roaming the room, literally draping herself over people with nary a word. Another teacher, without knowing my shoulder considerations and without asking, came from behind and yanked on my shoulder. Hands on hips, hands on thighs, hands somewhere you do not anticipate, the uninvited touch your only signal. Another walked around the room during the final resting pose and pulled on everyone's feet. Unannounced and uninvited. A suggestion: even if you are a talented yoga teacher, you can still be polite and respect personal space. So, to adjust or not to adjust? Let's keep considering.

**Command Central:** Consider that a key part of setting up a trauma-informed room is teachers staying on their mats. If walking around is not trauma-informed, what options are available to guide, to teach, and to adjust? Two relevant trauma-informed ideas to the rescue. One is that predictability and consistency build a sense of safety. The second is those who have experienced trauma often want to please and not want to draw attention to themselves. These facts give you four strong teaching options. 1) You have your voice. 2) You have yourself as a model. 3) You have the group. 4) And, you have someone's growing awareness of their bodily sensations. All these adjustments can happen from that predictable and consistent spot: your mat. Let's explore these options.

**All Together Now:** In a veteran's class, a fit younger woman was doing warrior two with her arms reversed. Faulty proprioception (knowing and sensing where you are in space) is not uncommon in trauma. Yet until then, I had not seen it in action. I said, "Okay, everyone, when you are ready, tap your front leg three times. Then raise that arm to shoulder height." She did the suggested tapping and proceeded back into her revolved-arm warrior. When I share that story in my workshops, I ask what a teacher should do next. I pause. Then I say, "Get on with your life." People laugh, but I am serious. If someone isn't in imminent danger, move on. I will share that after four weeks, she found the suggested warrior two. Someone can practice orienting in space by tapping the front leg three times. This tapping combines the sensory cues from the hand and leg with the visual cue of the front leg. Yoga indeed builds body awareness.

If someone has a front leg angling so that a bad habit or knee strain could happen, I say, "When you are ready, come back to standing." As a group, we begin anew. "If you like, tap your front leg. Then gently guide the leg so the knee isn't moving in." Yes, a lot of words, but I am modeling it, so it is easy to follow. And I exaggerate the movement to visually bring home the point. And, as always, it's a good reminder for everyone.

**Lookin' Good!** One key part of trauma recovery is reconnecting with physical sensations. As discussed in the language section, a clear, invitational cue (which does not include the word invite…) can keep the focus on how something *feels*, not on how it looks. "You may have a slight bend in your front leg, or perhaps today you bend the front leg in a different way. Find a way that feels strong today." Instead of adjustments based on how someone looks (a perfectly aligned 90-degree knee bend with the knee tracking over the middle toes), adjustments can be made based on how it feels today. As T.K.V. Desikachar says, "Yoga is not an external experience. … We do yoga only for ourselves. If you do not pay attention to ourselves in our practice, we cannot call it yoga" (Desikachar, 1995/1999).

## When Is Restorative Not Restorative?

Why is this question even in the section on safety? Because being trauma-informed is an approach, not a style of yoga, as are Hatha, Ashtanga, or vinyasa. Or restorative. Being trauma-informed can be a teaching guide for many styles of yoga. Restorative yoga may sound lovely. You may be spending time lying over bolsters to release muscle tension, lingering in calming twists, supporting your legs up a wall to get things moving in another direction, breathing easily, and thinking nice thoughts. You spend ten or more minutes in each position while listening to gentle nature sounds. So, again, why is restorative yoga discussed in the section on safety? For someone recovering from trauma, some important considerations follow.

**Stillness:** Styles of yoga that include long periods of not moving and of quiet can be triggering. Large body movements can allay anxiety. Stillness does not organize the attentional system. organize the attentional system.

**Peace and Quiet:** Long periods without a teacher's 'voice as a thread to safety' can create anxiety. If one of our physiological gauges for safety is the prosody (tone and rhythm) of someone's voice, periods of quiet deny us that key safety indicator. Someone may not feel comfortable closing their eyes, thus losing an opportunity to practice new self-regulation techniques. Closed eyes shut out one set of stimuli, freeing up attention to notice the breath and bodily sensations more fully. A talented yoga teacher shared that the teacher's voice was indeed a thread to safety for her in a restorative class. The teacher stopped talking during the last pose, creating ten minutes of quiet. "So, I could never fully relax at first because I was wondering, when will she say something again? This caused me more anxiety. I had a similar experience with yin yoga."

**Your Happy Place:** For some in trauma recovery, being left alone with their thoughts, nature music or not, can be unsettling. Their thoughts often are not conducive to restoring or resetting the nervous system.

**You Want Me to Do What?** Restorative body postures may feel vulnerable to those early in trauma recovery. For example, a supine bound angle pose, with or without a strap, can feel vulnerable. More vulnerable poses (Where are the hips? Where is the head?) are something to work toward when someone feels a stronger sense of safety in and control over their bodies. At that point, the pose can be empowering and not triggering.

**Changing of the Guard:** Moving to the next restorative pose often means reconfiguring the arrangement of the room. Such changes can lead to wondering: "Who will be next to me? How close? Where is the teacher? What is the teacher going to do to me?"

**What's in a Name?** There are talented yoga teachers who never mention trauma but clearly teach with an awareness of safety, empowerment, and simplicity. Conversely, a class with a peaceful sounding name doesn't make it or the teacher trauma-informed. Chapter 5 discusses the importance of making responsible referrals and ways to empower someone to find trauma-informed teachers (p. 94).

## Supporting Empowerment

### Word Choice – It's the Little Things

Ideas on the power of word choice are discussed in the chapters on language and on the breath. Let's consider why word choice directly affects both planning and teaching trauma-informed yoga, whether a a short break or a full practice.

**One Little Word:** I started including the word *today* in breathwork. I then started using it in other parts of the practice as well. *Today* highlights the time is now, not yesterday. And something might be different tomorrow.

**Another Little Word:** Why do I teach, 'Find a *New* Stretch'? It introduces something new within the safety of familiar breathwork and movement. "Perhaps move in a way to create a *new* stretch." Or "Give yourself a few moments to find a *new* stretch. You can follow me, or you can find your own *new* stretches today." Leaving someone adrift without an idea or your voice to follow may yank away your gentle guidance and the opportunity to widen their window of tolerance.

**Delete:** You may want to consider hitting the delete button on the word *just.* "If you can't touch the floor, *just* put your hands above your knees" can become: "When you are ready, place your hand above your knee. This may be your stretch today, or you may want to move your hand down your leg." The word *just* minimizes or negatively qualifies most things.

**Power Up:** I teach many with physical or emotional challenges. One day while teaching a warrior two flow I said, "Warrior two is a power pose. If you like, practice it in a way that feels strong today." Including at least one noted power pose or variation provides someone with opportunities to feel strong today. From children in low-income schools, to refugees and immigrants, and to veterans, an overwhelming favorite is tree pose. What reasons occur to you? I thought of five. 1) Tree pose uses large muscles in the legs and the core. Someone can *feel* their body. 2) Someone may notice weekly progress, empowered by feeling strength building and a sense of mastery. 3) The cue that "You can put your foot down anytime, you are never stuck," gives an opportunity to *feel* not being stuck and to practice choice. 4) Trying to 'find your balance' can clear one's mind of other thoughts. It focuses attention, so it can be a quick mental reset. 5) The second side of tree pose is playful. "If you like, move your arms in a way that makes you smile." Again, play allows someone to explore new actions and outcomes within the safety of something known. And again (and again), none of these reasons is explained. 'Show, Don't Tell.'

## The Building Blocks of Choice

Why is choice so important in a trauma-informed approach? Choice sets the stage for personal growth and empowerment. Perhaps today is a day to try something new, to take effective action. As Judith Herman, MD, said in her foundational book, *Trauma and Recovery*: "The guiding principle of recovery is restoring a sense of power and control to the survivor" (Herman, 1997). Choice is empowering, until it's not. Something is not empowering when it overwhelms or distracts or both. A woman with two service dogs on her mat said as I was blathering on about options, "Don't give me any more choices. I can't handle that today." I was glad someone finally stopped me. Note that too many choices are a clear example of too much of a good thing. 'More is not better, more is confusing'. So, let's start with the most basic of choices and build from there.

**One Action:** David Emerson's phrases "when you are ready" and "if you like" denote simple choices (Emerson and Hopper, 2011). A person can decide when they are ready or if they want to do this one thing. "If you like, put one or both hands over your heart." You can pause and repeat it, giving people a chance to process what you have said without losing the thread of your voice. Someone told me after class that they didn't want to put their hands over their heart today, so they didn't. Of note was that she wanted to share this observation.

'Small choices. Small points of awareness Small movements toward trauma recovery'.

**Two Actions:** You offer two simple choices. "Anything we do standing, you can do seated. You can always find ways to breathe and move with me." Leaving it open-ended supports someone finding their way. If you stand, then sit, then stand again, you may leave someone adrift, watching and wondering what to do. Another example: "Today you may like to take your hand off the chair to strengthen core muscles. Or you may keep your hand on the chair to focus on the stretch. 'Different days, different stretches'." This choice also provides the opportunity to experience personal growth as choices change.

**A Matter of Degree:** In these cues, notice how someone can easily explore different degrees of movement along the same continuum. "The suggestion is to lift one arm, either

to the side or overhead. If it is comfortable today, arc that arm over your head. If you like, stretch your fingers wide." Another example: "When you are ready, find *new* things to stretch. Today you might like to move with me, or you might move in your own way." I keep cueing breathwork and movement in a simple flow, with 'my voice as a thread to safety'. The simple choice continuum reinforces that it's their practice and that I support exploring different ways of practicing. I have been in classes in which the teacher was visibly annoyed when instructions were not followed.

## Of Boundaries and Personal Growth

Why is failing to articulate clear boundaries a missed opportunity? Creating a verbal boundary gives someone control as they decide if three times is 'comfortable for you today'. "Okay, she said we can practice this flow three times. But we can come out of it anytime. We are never stuck. She said that." Such simple techniques can support widening the window of tolerance, a key to part of developing resiliency skills. 'Teach to Empower'.

## Knowledge Is Power

A guide to what information would be helpful is the simple question: is this information empowering or overwhelming? As I iterated my trauma-informed teaching, I thought offering one body-based benefit for each pose could be empowering. "Tree pose can build core muscles," or "Tree pose can improve balance." I continue to notice the positive effect in facial expressions. Do I mention the laundry list of core muscles and what they do? I do not. Offering one point of information also can turn a directive into a choice. "Don't put your foot on your knee," can become, "Pressing your foot on the knee puts extra pressure on your knee joint." You have empowered someone to protect their knee with one simple, nondirective fact. 'More is not better, ...' well, you know the rest.

## Normalize and Set Up for Success

Most of us do not like to do things that make us feel inadequate or weak. Normalizing variations is a way to set someone up for success. Normalizing means, quite literally, showing how something is normal, not indicative of weakness or lacking talent or ability. Some who have experienced trauma already feel shame and guilt. A trauma-informed teacher is inclusive, nonjudgmental, and supportive. The following examples normalize different ways to practice yoga. A reason follows each and is only for your information. It is in keeping with the theme of this book: 'Be informed and be inspired'.

- **Cue:** "Anything that we do standing you can do seated or even lying down. Find a way to breathe and move that is comfortable for you today."

**Reason:** Someone may find sitting painful. Once an older veteran did an entire hour of yoga lying on a table.

- **Cue:** "Today may be a day to move in a *new* way. Part of your practice is finding what you need today."

**Reason:** This cue can build a sense of time, widen the window of tolerance, and foster some body awareness. Encouraging someone to notice what they need today is not only grounding but also empowering. The message is someone is both worthy and capable of creating a practice that meets their needs today, which may include stress or pain management.

- **Cue:** "The benefit comes from finding a better way to move, not in how much you stretch."

**Reason:** A thought from Moshe Feldenkrais, PhD, a trained physicist who then devoted his life and brilliance to body-based healing, is there isn't a right way to move, there is a better way to move (Feldenkrais, 1981/2019). For some, large movements are uncomfortable or simply not possible. This advice can help someone with pain or energy challenges feel engaged while practicing with small movements. You also are letting everyone know someone moving in a different way is 'finding that better way to move'.

- **Cue**: "Even small stretches have benefits."

**Reason:** Moshe Feldenkrais, also one of the first neuroplasticians, believed that the brain rewired more quickly as we practiced small, slow movements (Feldenkrais, 1972/1977). I have had many tell me that thinking about their practice in this way changed it from, "I can't do yoga," to "Oh, I can do this – I can move in a way that feels good and that has benefit."

- **Cue**: "If you have stronger muscles, you can benefit from stretching. If you are more flexible, you may benefit from strengthening. Yoga offers both."

**Reason:** It can be empowering to know that yoga builds both muscle and flexibility. Sharing this fact normalizes the variations in the room.

## Maintaining Simplicity

'Trust the Yoga' and 'Show, Don't Tell' are introduced in Chapter 2. These trauma-informed ideas can simplify both how you plan and how you teach. As Steve Jobs is credited with saying: "'Focus and simplicity' has been one of my mantras. Simple can be harder than complex … But it's worth it in the end because once you get there, you can move mountains." Or perhaps you can be instrumental in someone's trauma recovery.

A GreenTREE Yoga® certified yoga teacher shared a comment from a woman at the county jail (thank you, Mariann!).

In Warrior I, I suggested looking forward or looking up. When we gently stepped back to mountain pose, a woman said, with tears rolling down her face, 'Oh my gosh, I just realized, standing in this pose, looking up to the ceiling, that I have been making myself small for other people's benefit, so they will feel comfortable around me. I don't take up space in the world and I have been doing that for a very long time, it just hit me like a ton of bricks.'

Simple teaching supported this woman's yoga experience by giving her the mental space to think and to feel. Let's look at how to access the power of teaching simply by considering options that keep cues free of the clutter of explanations and words.

## Keeping It Simple

Literal and body-based cues simplify understanding. "Reach for the sky as you open the side body," can become: "As you stretch your arm over your head, notice where you feel the stretch." Another path to keeping it simple is thoughtful planning. For example, in teaching warrior two, if you planned your one alignment cue to be rolling to the baby-toe edge of the back foot (to protect the knee joint), then plan rolling to the inside/outside edges of the feet in your beginning wide-legged add-on pose (p. 234 (a)–(c)). Thoughtful planning gives less new information to process, so someone might think, "Oh, okay, I know this. We did this." In keeping with the idea that 'More is not better, more is confusing', perhaps offer no more than one alignment and one physical benefit for each pose.

## Consistent Phrasing

Why is consistent phrasing a strong addition to your teaching plan? Again (and again), it allows you to keep the thread of your voice going without giving new information to process. And you are giving someone time to experience what you are suggesting.

**Let's Practice Prasarita Padottanasana:** While Sanskrit words may be fun to say, the words do not support keeping it simple or giving it (verbal part of the brain) a rest. However, consistently naming a pose allows for recognition. When you say tree pose, someone may be getting set up for the pose before you cue it, also building some sense of mastery. Someone also can ask about a pose later or to do it at home. Recognition is the reason every pose and breath in this book is named, for example 'Tip-to-Toe' stretch or the 'Anytime, Anywhere Breath'. Your teaching stays consistent and predictable.

"Oh, I know this," can be a thought or *feeling* when you say, "Let's get set up for 'Kitchen Stretch.'"

**Reach for the Sky:** Perhaps play along and practice this cue while reading it aloud: "When you are ready, reach one hand toward the ceiling and spread your fingers. Then, if you like, stretch your other arm up high and move your fingers as wide apart as you can." The cues are literal and body-based: reach, stretch, hand, arm, fingers, ceiling. So, now what's the problem? It might seem picky, but it is not. It's about consistently giving it a rest. It's about keeping wording simple, so more mental energy (yes, thinking literally takes energy) is available to notice both the breath and bodily sensations. Let's try again. If you are still playing along, practice these cues while reading them aloud. 1) "When you are ready, reach one hand toward the ceiling and spread your fingers. Then stretch your other arm up high and move your fingers as wide apart as you can. When you are ready, release your arms." Then: 2) "When you are ready, stretch one arm overhead, fingers stretched wide. Then stretch your other arm overhead, fingers stretched wide." What did you notice? The same wording makes it easier to understand and easier to teach.

## Mixing It Up without Getting Mixed Up

You are predictable. You are consistent. Are you boring? Adding variations can spice it up and keep someone engaged and curious. But note that a variation is not the same as offering more options. You can do it seated on the floor, seated in a chair, you can do it standing on your mat, you can do it standing near a wall, you can do it standing on one leg, you can do it … well, you get the idea. Many options mean many words and ideas to process. Again, you want to give someone time to understand your suggestion, to find their way to do the pose, and to notice the breath and the bodily sensations. Extra verbal tasks can steal that time.

A Vietnam veteran, who'd been coming to my class for four years, told me that what he liked about my class was that he never knew what I was going to do next. The other teacher was boring, always the same thing, he noted. At first, this struck me as curious, since I have the same general outline for the classes. But then I realized he was focusing on the different ways in which I taught the same poses. To him, that kept it fresh. Proof that the structure with slight variation can work.

Chapter 1 discusses the science of how stress impairs learning. Two ideas can keep your teaching trauma-informed. The first is that studies show voluntary attention increases learning. The teaching suggestion is to build voluntary attention through simple choice. The second idea is researchers for Blue's Clues (educational television) found that children learn new things better from a base of the familiar (Crawly et al., 1999). Therefore, the teaching suggestion is to introduce variations when someone is familiar with finding a way to do the pose "that is comfortable for you today." Here are two ideas that avoid a confusing laundry list of options.

1) **A slight change** to the cue works from that familiar base. On the third shoulder say, "If you like, move even more slowly now." Or, "If you like, stop the roll halfway down. Hold the stretch but not your breath … hold the stretch but not your breath. Let's practice 2 more breaths here. Feel the breath in … Feel the breath out." (*Say 2 times slowly.*)

2) **A variation on the second side** of a pose can keep attention while keeping it simple. For example, "As we do tree pose on this side, perhaps stretch one or both arms overhead, fingers stretched wide." Or "On this side, the suggestion is to move your arms in a *new* way if you like." Acknowledging the change in cueing *before* you teach it maintains consistency and predictability. "Yael always tells us when something changes," can be someone's thought or *feeling*. You can build a sense of curiosity without losing that safe base of the familiar. If these ideas make sense, you will find more variations both for breathwork in Chapter 7 and for the practice sequences in Chapter 11. Your clipboard plan can include variation ideas.

Now let's take these considerations of *why* planning what you say and do (or don't say and do) in the physical practice is important and look at *how* to plan a yoga practice so someone might feel what an Afghani refugee community leader shared after our class: "Peace of mind … I feel some peace."

**********

**To Recap:** There are many considerations before making the all-important teaching plan. If you want to use trauma-informed yoga to organize the attentional system and help someone to focus and to learn, give yourself the time to carefully read (or reread) this chapter. You can organize your thoughts on *why* simple breathwork and movement, your pacing, and your use of language, can empower someone to widen their window of tolerance. The ideas in this chapter set a firm foundation for the next chapter: *how* to plan and to teach your trauma-informed practice. 'Be informed and be inspired'.

## References

Crawley, A., et al. (1999). Effects of Repeated Exposure of Single Episode of Blue's Clues. *Journal of Educational Psychology*, 91, 630–637.

Desikachar, T. K. V. (1995/1999). *The Heart of Yoga: Developing a Personal Practice.* Rochester, VT: Inner Traditions, p. 23.

Emerson, David and Hopper, Elizabeth. (2011). *Overcoming Trauma Through Yoga.* Berkeley, CA: North Atlantic Books, p. 121.

Feldenkrais, Moshe. (1972/1977). *Awareness Through Movement.* New York: Harper One, pp. 36–37.

Feldenkrais, Moshe. (1981/2019). *The Elusive Obvious: The Convergence of Movement, Neuroplasticity and Mental Health.* Berkley, CA: North Atlantic Books, pp. 92–93.

Herman, Judith. (1997). *Trauma and Recovery.* New York: Basic Books, p. 160.

Levine, Peter. (2010). *In An Unspoken Voice.* Berkeley, CA: North Atlantic Books, p. 79.

NICABM #2. *When Mindfulness Will (and Won't) Work for Treating Trauma with Bessel van der Kolk, MD.*

Rizzolatti, Giacomo, et al. (2004). The Mirror-Neuron System. *Annual Review of Neuroscience*, 27, 169–192.

Ogden, Pat. (2006). *Trauma and the Body.* New York: W. W. Norton and Company, p. 273.

Van der Kolk, Bessel A. (2015). *The Body Keeps the Score: Brain, Mind, and Body in the Healing of Trauma.* New York: Penguin Publishing.

# 9
# Steps to Creating Your Practice

## Step One: A Plan Can ...

### How to Not 'End Up Someplace Else'

As the baseball coach Yogi Berra is credited with saying, "If you don't know where you are going, you will end up someplace else." Planning a strong practice will support your efforts to not end up someplace else.

- **Confidence:** You will be organized and feel more confident, which will come across in your voice and add to the sense of safety in the room.
- **Pacing:** You will not be rushed, a stressed feeling that can be transmitted to your students. You also will not end up with too much time, grabbing for filler poses that are not part of the plan.
- **Consistency:** Your class will be predictable and consistent, also building a feeling of safety.
- **Attention:** You can focus on your students, clients, or patients without the distraction of deciding what to do next. A teacher told me that having a plan made her class flow, so she could pay attention to her word choice and to noticing the class needs.

### How Long Is Long Enough?

People continue to be happily surprised when I offer that even a few minutes of yoga can have a positive effect in real-time. One of the many strengths of yoga is its inherent flexibility. Class length is determined by time constraints, obviously, but also by the needs of the participants. Sometimes shorter classes or yoga breaks are a better fit for someone with sleep or pain challenges. Be confident that the key to a successful teaching experience is good planning and not length of time.

DOI: 10.4324/9781003308836-12

**Ways to Extend a Practice:** You look at the time and realize that you have an extra ten minutes. Does your clipboard plan include what to do with extra time? Saying, "Let's do three shoulder stretches again," makes the practice consistent. The practice sequences and the clipboard notes include suggestions on ways to smoothly extend these practices (Chapter 11). We will circle back to the power of clipboards.

**Group Connection.** You also can ask, "Is there a breath or stretch you'd like to do again? Let's practice two suggestions." Putting a boundary on the number of suggestions keeps the practice predictable. Someone may say, "Let's do 'Kitchen Stretch' again." And someone may add, "Oh, I love that one." Connections made.

**Ways Not to Extend a Practice:** If you allot 15 minutes for the 'Final Stretch' all guided by your voice, create consistency by keeping that schedule. A number of people mentioned that teachers adding extra quiet time as filler created feelings of stress.

## Adapting for Pain and Differing Abilities

None of the suggestions in this book is medical advice. This section offers adaptations for physical, emotional, and mental considerations, as well as pain. As with any trauma-informed practice, your role is to guide opportunities to reconnect with physical sensations and to empower someone to practice self-regulation. You have succeeded if someone can create the practice they need today. It's a bonus if later they practice or share ideas on self-regulation.

Books have been written on sharing yoga with specific populations, and rightly so. But a laundry list of adaptations will miss the mark. You may not know everyone's concerns. As you demonstrate the laundry list, you break the flow of the class and instead become a distraction. A common question is how to teach to a group with mixed or differing needs. My advice is to focus on teaching to empower everyone to find their own way, an approach that also takes pressure off you. I have taught classes that included someone on oxygen with a walker and someone who ran 10 Ks. If you are okay with it, they will be too. 'Teach to Empower'.

**Repetition:** It is helpful to find trauma-informed cues that resonate with you and use them often. People share that hearing these cues repeated gave them the confidence to try different things. Tables 11.1, 11.2, and 11.3 list suggested phrases and times to use them.

**Inclusivity:** If someone is in a wheelchair or chooses to sit down, include them in your cueing. Everyone should *feel* seen and *feel* a part of the group.

"When you are ready, put your hands on on the sides of your chair or your hips ." Putting the seated cue first is practicing inclusivity and indicates you support someone taking a seat at any time. "When you are ready, gently move from side to side. Feel yourself shift as you are sitting or shifting on your feet."

**Back Pain:** Many in my classes, including veterans, clinicians, refugees, and the incarcerated, have back pain. Books have been written on yoga for back pain. Given the overlap between trauma and pain, it seems a lost opportunity not to teach pain management in a trauma-informed way. How can yoga help manage back pain? The short answer is that medical providers often suggest gentle stretching and various breathing techniques to decrease mental and physical stress, as well as pain. My short answer is to follow the protocols outlined in this book. My much longer answer is in my book *Trauma-informed Yoga for Pain Management: A Practical Manual for Simple Stretching, Gentle Strengthening, and Mindful Breathing* (2024).

**Injuries:** I have taught those with diverse injuries: healing broken bones (shoulder/foot/arm/wrist/leg), torn rotator cuffs, various back conditions or injuries, and hip and knee replacements. Begin with gentle movements to stretch the areas around the injury, often tight from disuse. Teach breathwork to lower physical, emotional, and mental stress, which often causes tight muscles and increased pain. Create balanced stretching and strengthening opportunities to maintain healthy spinal and hip alignment as someone heals. I learned a valuable insight from a long-time participant who continued in our class after she had broken her leg. I kept stopping to show chair adaptations. She laughed, "I can figure it out, don't worry." And she did. She then added, "You know, I did that breathing we learned on the way to the hospital."

**Fibromyalgia, Rheumatoid Arthritis (RA), and other Pain Issues:** An overactive immune system, not uncommon in trauma, can lead to painful and exhausting immune disorders. I taught a retired lawyer with a lifetime of complex traumas, an admitted type-A personality, also with fibromyalgia, and several back/neck issues from four car accidents. She shared that it took many weeks, but she finally believed moving even a centimeter had benefits. She believed it because she had felt it. I taught several women with fibromyalgia and RA. Watching them struggle to make a fist inspired me to adapt 'Fist Breathing' ('Open and Close Breath') to empower those with gnarled hands or painful fingers. The adaptation also builds body awareness in everyone (p. 127).

**Larger Bodies:** Yoga can be accessible to all shapes and sizes. Be aware such words as weight and belly may cause discomfort. Choose poses that do not create feelings of failure. In some larger bodies, deep twists or lying on the stomach may not feel empowering. Moving from standing to the floor and back again may also be challenging and make someone feel unsuccessful. I encourage you to use this guide: your common sense.

**Paralysis:** Consider the case of a man in his 40s, paralyzed from the chest down in a snowboarding accident and still in the hospital. His therapist wanted to do a 30-minute yoga practice to help with trauma and pain. My advice was to work with what you have: hands, fingers, head, shoulders, and the breath. He taught a lot of breathwork using hands and finger movements. He did the shoulder exercises outlined in the practice sequences. An additional tool was to work with muscle tonus (partial contraction of the muscle or resistance to stretch) and brain maps. Norman Doidge, MD, discusses this interesting feature of the brain: thoughts can activate the brain maps and stimulate muscle tonus (Doidge, 2015). Or quite simply, visualizing movements can have physical benefits. Sometimes his wife or other family participated, an opportunity to teach tools for use at home. His wife said, "I think I just breathed more than I have all day." Someone else shared, "I felt energy shooting from my hand during 'The Wave Breath.'" These remote classes were by phone. 'Trust the Yoga'.

**Traumatic Brain Injury (TBI):** I worked with an older veteran who, based on my observations alone, had challenges processing words to put into physical movements. As we were doing fist motions in warrior two, she blurted out, "This feels amazing!" In 'Final Stretch', she did nothing I suggested but moved in her own way. She sat up at the end and again blurted out, "This felt wonderful to me!" Later I found out she had a TBI diagnosis. Someone can indeed create their own practice. She was a part of our yoga group for many months.

**Autism:** Autism spectrum disorder (ASD) ranges from high-to-low-functioning. A rule of thumb is to follow your trauma-informed protocol. A 19-year-old woman was no longer able to remain in her home, but her parents wanted some yoga classes before she moved. The teacher designed a practice based on the woman's interest in nursery rhymes. They played her favorite calming music in the background. The teacher got into this young woman's world as best she could. She focused on breaths with hand pressure (fist breathing, arm wraps) and rocking poses with a lot of grounding opportunities. Yoga is flexible. My book on art and yoga for differing needs and autism has many more ideas (Calhoun, 2025).

**Hearing or Visual Impairment:** To review, mammals use the social engagement system (features of the voice and facial expressions) to gauge safety. Be confident by using trauma-informed protocols, you have it covered. A visually impaired veteran emailed me years later, saying that I probably didn't remember her, but she had such fond memories of our class. "I can still hear your voice. You could put me to sleep."

## Connect the Dots

Obviously, there are many teaching situations. These ideas in this chapter may inspire your confidence in using the GreenTREE Yoga® Approach as a versatile teaching tool. A plan can help connect the dots. Given that we are over 60 percent water, moving in a fluid way seems natural. You can create that embodied opportunity to flow. Planning can keep a flow in your practice and avoid disruptions. "Now we will do one more standing balance before we take a seat," creates a predictable connection. "If you like, practice a long breath in … As YOU breathe out, sit in a way that feels comfortable for you today," creates a connection using simple breathwork and movement. The takeaway is to create opportunities to keep someone engaged and present (grounded) using a simple flow of breathwork and movement.

**Chatting:** Whether working with a group or an individual, nervous chatter can break your flow. You respectfully can set those boundaries. "Let's talk after class, now let's focus on our practice." Page 74 has more suggestions.

**Watch Me:** It is worth another mention. If you pause to demonstrate options, you have broken the flow with disjointed actions as you sit, stand, or lie down. Simple, clear guidance is enough: "Anything we do standing you can do seated or lying down. You can always find comfortable ways to breathe and to move with me." In all my years of teaching, I have never observed someone at a loss for what to do. And remember, you do not know what will work today. Someone may not know until they try. 'Teach to Empower'.

## Your Planning Checklist: A Quick Review

Why is this book filled with quick reviews? Because key ideas are worth repeating as they frame each of the strategies for creating a trauma-informed practice. Someone with a PTSD diagnosis wrote in her class evaluation, "I feel like I can handle anything now on the drive home."

Another reason to plan is a comment from a trauma therapist after her 90-minute private session. She arrived and announced she could not feel her body. She really didn't think this would help, but *her* therapist thought she should try. After 'Final Stretch', she sat up and said, "I was fully present. This was amazing. Before this class I felt like I was in the shower with a raincoat on. After the class I felt like the raincoat had come off and could feel the warm shower." She then repeated the whole comment, as it seemed to surprise her. What special practice had I planned? I used the practices included in Chapter 11. As you plan, consider this checklist:

**Safety:** Perhaps review the ideas outlined in Chapters 3 and 4 on how to create a sense of safety in the room. Remember, if someone does not feel safe, learning new ways of processing and responding to perceived threats is difficult. 'It's body physiology'.

**Empowerment:** Creating opportunities to empower is a key part of the planning process. Is your language empowering? Are you offering simple choices? 'Small choices. Small points of awareness. Small movements toward trauma recovery'.

**Simplicity:** It literally takes energy to think. A helpful trauma-informed guide can be 'Simple to do. Simple to understand'.

**The Power of the Clipboard:** Most will acknowledge the shift to trauma-informed teaching has many moving parts. Using a clipboard can simplify your life. This sign of strong teaching also indicates you care about what you are offering, you are organized, and you have given thought to someone's needs. Perhaps reread that last sentence because clipboards give many positive messages. A single page with two columns placed where you glance at it as you teach can include: 1) Outline of the class – beginning, middle, and closing, including today's breathwork; 2) Outline three or four key phrases to use/repeat; and 3) Ways to adjust for time (too much, too little). Again, using a clipboard can build confidence in your teaching abilities – confidence for you and for your students, clients, or patients. Clipboard sheets are in Appendix C: Supplemental Resources.

## The Last Piece of the Planning Puzzle

You can prepare a wonderful trauma-informed yoga practice, but there remains another piece to the planning puzzle. People need to come. If you are teaching in a residential facility, usually activities are scheduled. People still may need to sign up. For many, trying a new activity can be stressful and outside their windows of tolerance. How do you support trying something outside of someone's comfort zone? I will share some ideas.

**Hear All About It!** A simple flyer to the staff person organizing the class provides a good introduction (Appendix C: Supplemental Resources). Choose the name of your class with awareness of the group. Sometimes using the word trauma in the name deters someone who does not want to self-identify as having had trauma. Or, someone may think the class includes more trauma talk therapy. Be mindful of including possible trigger words in the name. You may want to find less reactive words than *relax* and *body*. With one older group, I called the class 'Simple Stretching and Breathing'. For other classes, since referrals came with clinical diagnoses of PTSD or military sexual trauma, the class was 'Trauma-informed Yoga'. With refugee and prison groups, I do not put trauma in the class name. As with all things trauma-informed, make a conscious decision on your group needs. One size does not fit all.

**Of Boundaries and Choice:** Offering a class series of four to six weeks can be helpful. Someone may not feel trapped or overwhelmed with a set time boundary. It also gives them the opportunity to say, "I am sorry I can't help you out, I have this class on Tuesdays." If you plan to run the class for longer, you can present another round of sign-up opportunities. Choosing to attend can be empowering, a step in "the pleasure of completed action," as Pierre Janet, MD, said over a hundred years ago.

**Who Is This?** Where appropriate, it is good practice to call participants as an introduction and to answer any questions. When I taught veterans, I quickly realized that the well-intended office person had many other calls to make and could not answer questions. Taking over the task of calling was time well spent as I was able to connect and to allay concerns. Yes, the class is for all abilities. Yes, you can come to the class, and if it is not a good fit, you can leave anytime. Yes, simply get up and leave, it is not a problem. No, you do not need special clothes or to bring a yoga mat. Yes, you certainly can bring someone with you (but not a child). No, they do not have to be a veteran. I cannot tell you how many times I have heard, "Well, you said …" And, indeed, I had.

**Points of Connection Continued:** Another good practice can be text reminders. For morning classes, I have found the night before works well. For afternoon or evening classes, a same day morning text is usually much appreciated. I have often heard, "Oh, I totally spaced on the class until I got your text this morning, thank you." As I have mentioned, this texting sets the stage for future points of connection as most people keep in touch and enjoy the seasonal photos I often include.

As a courtesy, always ask if someone would like a reminder text. Some people thank me, but say they have a calendar. One older man told me that he was so nervous on Wednesdays wondering when I was going to text. I told him that was fine, I wouldn't text anymore. He continued, saying he needed to explain. I told him that was not necessary. He pressed on, saying I did not understand, all his life he had never stood up for himself. So now he wanted me to know. One younger veteran texted me back, "I am so grateful for your texts. At least I know someone knows I am out here." And as always, be aware of personal boundaries, including your own.

## Step Two: Sequencing the Yoga Practice

What are the three guiding principles for sequencing a trauma-informed yoga practice? You already may have answered the question. A sequence has a predictable order based on building safety, supporting empowerment, and maintaining simplicity. A predictable order means the class has a beginning, a middle, and an end. I think of it as a sequencing wave, the ebb and flow, of body-based yoga. You start slowly with grounding, work toward appropriately challenging flows and poses, and end with more grounding. I have heard the last ten minutes of a practice described as giving the clay time to set or the nervous system a chance to process what you have just done. Each part of the practice adds to the synergy of breathwork and movement.

### Begin at the Beginning

As mentioned before, musing about the benefits of yoga or your qualifications is telling, not showing. A stronger start to your class is embracing your role as a guide for grounding. But what if someone is new, don't they need to be filled in? It took me many wordy attempts, but I settled on: "Welcome, find an open spot. Always breathe and move in a way that is comfortable to you today." It also serves as a nice reminder to everyone as well. 'Trust the Yoga'.

**Setting an Intention:** Some teachers begin class by setting an intention. I have found that first offering five minutes of simple breathing and movement is better preparation for setting an intention, a verbal function. The next section outlines many grounding exercises with which to begin. Simplicity is the guide. "You may like to set an intention for your practice today. It may be the reason that you joined us today. Or perhaps today your intention is to notice a stretch that feels comfortable to you." I give only two suggestions. It is not helpful for someone to think, "I can't even think of an intention, I shouldn't even be here." It's also not helpful for someone to feel overwhelmed by choices. 'Teach to Empower'.

## Grounding – It Never Gets Old

To ground is from the old English root *grund*, meaning the bottom or the foundation. Having a firm foundation from which to meet the events of the day seems a worthy intention. A body-based yoga practice offers many ways to provide grounding guidance throughout the practice: set the opening tone for your class; pause to ground between poses; or practice grounding tools when you notice someone becoming distracted or disconnected (dissociated). These body-based ideas use rhythmic breathwork and movements (both subtle and large) to ground. All can be adapted to sitting, standing, and lying down. These following build on the simple breathwork in Chapter 7. Let's consider many simple ways to offer grounding guidance throughout the yoga practice or during a clinical or health care session.

**A Matched Set – the Breath and the Hands/Feet:** Use throughout the practice. Because you are doing the yoga together, extra words to explain every movement are unnecessary. 'Simple to understand. Simple to do'.

- **The Feet.** Changing the pressure on the feet sends new sensory signals to the brain and can build body awareness. A yoga teacher shared what she noticed about my practice was she could not stop wondering if I would remember to do the other side. I now start the cues with, "We always do both sides." You might like to stand now and experience the these simple grounding opportunities.

  1) **To experience a change of body position:** "When you are ready, step toward the back of your mat." Or "If you like, move your feet in some way." Or "If you like, move one foot off the mat." Or "Move one foot so the baby toe is off the mat and the big toe is on the mat."
  2) **To experience changes in pressure:** "When you are ready, step your feet apart and roll from the inside to the outside edges of your feet." Or "If you like, lift one heel and press on your toes, then lift the other heel and press on your toes." Or "As YOU breathe in, press down on your big toes ... as YOU breathe out, release."
  3) **To experience finding balance:** "When you are ready, lift (or stretch) all your toes in a comfortable way." Or "If you like, as YOU breathe in, shift forward, heels may lift ... as YOU breathe out, shift back, heels release."

Well, you get the idea. Simple to do, simple for you to remember: move the feet.

- **The Hands.** As a reminder of Iyengar's wisdom that yoga needs to be experienced, perhaps give yourself a few moments to do each of the following now. Press gently on your fingertips; tap your hands firmly on your legs; hold the sides of the chair; press your hands on your hips; and lift your arms overhead with fingertips pressing. Again, you get the idea. You can vary the press (gentle or firm) and vary the parts of the hands used (fingertips, palms, fingers, or the entire hand). I have had many comments that "the fingertips pressing on my legs felt so good." Simple to do, simple for you to remember: create pressure on the hands.

**Opportunity Knocks:** There are more opportunities to provide grounding guidance.

- **The Lips.** Wait, what? Does the cue 'smack the lips' or 'lick the lips' sound trauma-informed? How do we include the lips, brimming with sensory receptors, in a trauma-informed way? This simple cue met my teaching intention, and you may think of others. "As YOU are ready, feel your breath in … as YOU are ready, breathe out as if through a straw." Someone may feel the breath on their pursed lips, building both breath and body awareness while avoiding trigger words.
- **Where am I?** Well, more specifically, where is my arm? This awareness of where you presently are in space by sensing location and movement is called proprioception. In trauma, diminished function is not uncommon. One way to help reactivate this GPS of the brain (the posterior cingulate) is to cue looking at your hands as you move or as you stretch your fingers wide.
- **Where's the Stretch?** A common question is, "Where should I feel this?" "You should feel it in your upper back," is a lost grounding opportunity. Someone should notice what they notice, not what you tell them. "You should feel the stretch in your hamstrings," can become: "Notice where you feel the stretch. Different days, different stretches." "You will feel a deep stretch on your side when you lift your arm," can become: "Notice if the stretch changes as you lift your arm." One day I said, "Notice where you feel the stretch." An older woman with a great attitude and a good bit of trauma said out loud, "Okay, I know it's in here somewhere." When we did the other side, she sounded surprised as she blurted, "Oh, there it is, there it is!"

- **Have a Heart.** Many have told me how they love this suggestion, and how surprised they are at how it feels. "If you like, put one or both hands over your heart. When you feel your heart beating … when you feel your heart beating, press down on your fingertips."
- **Slow Your Roll.** Consciously regulating the speed at which we move happens in the present. Consider how these cues build body awareness and a sense of control. "If you like, move your leg even more slowly from side to side." Or "When you are ready, circle the other way, perhaps even more slowly."
- **Find Your Rhythm.** Noticing the rhythm of your breathing and movement happens in the present. 'Find your own rhythm' can be a life-affirming suggestion as it uses both breath and movement to ground. Opportunities to practice 'finding your own rhythm' are in the scripts for seated twists and wide-legged add-ons (pp. 222/226/226–227).
- **Fill in the Blank.** To make this your own, the 'Show, Don't Tell' pattern for creating grounding opportunities is first to suggest noticing a physical sensation followed by a small movement acknowledging to yourself that you noticed. "When you notice the muscles in your arms working … when you notice the muscles in your arms working, press down on your toes." Then later a slight cue change can keep someone engaged and curious.

**It's Beyond Me:** We are bombarded with sensory signals, but healthy brains have well-tuned filtering systems, so we are not overwhelmed. As discussed in Chapter 1, the ability to process sensory input from within ourselves (I feel my muscles working, I feel warm, I feel my heart beating) is called interoception. We also receive large sets of sensory inputs from outside of the physical self, a process aptly named exteroception. How can this physiological fact be used to your teaching advantage? To build on the ideas in Chapter 3, noticing various external cues and pairing that awareness with subtle body movements can be used as grounding guides.

- **Sight.** Turning the centerpiece: "If you like, look at the flowers in the center of our circle. Perhaps notice a new color or shape. Then, tap your hand on your leg."
- **Sound:** "If you like, notice a new sound in the room. If there are no new sounds, notice that. Then, wiggle the fingers on one hand."
- **Touch.** "If you like, pick up the rock or shell from your mat and without looking at it, move it in your hand. Now if you like, gently close your fingers around it."

- **Smell.** "If you like, pick up the sprig of herb from the front of your mat. Does the smell change if you rub the leaves?"
- **Taste.** Sharing food, either before or after the practice, is a way to build a sense of safety and community, as well as to ground.

## The Middle: Creating Sequences That Flow

> I always come into this class so stressed. This class really calms me down. It makes me stretch in other areas of my life. I try it, I pull back, I try it, I pull back.
>
> ~ Rachel, a member of our Warrior Renew (military sexual trauma) class.

**The Building Blocks of the Practice Sequences:** These practice sequences are based on these three building blocks: building safety, supporting empowerment, and maintaining simplicity.

1. **Building Safety:** Consistency builds a sense of safety as someone knows what is coming next. "When you are ready, stand behind your chair," prompted a young veteran, recently back from Afghanistan, to ask while he was moving, "Oh, oh, are we going to do pyramid pose or tree pose?" It was his third class. Consistency creates a base of the familiar, creating an opportunity to add something new within a context of the known.
2. **Supporting Empowerment:** Consistency fosters empowerment as someone can notice improvement and changes from week to week. A young veteran who for months had walked from the residential substance abuse facility, said, "Did you see my tree pose today? Did you see my tree pose?" It was clearly important to him that I had, so I said, "Yes, it looked as though you felt strong today." I was surprised when a woman in the military sexual trauma class blurted out, "Whoa, I can really feel my inner thighs stretch. I like that stretch."
3. **Maintaining Simplicity:** Consistent sequences allow you to keep it simple. Bessel van der Kolk notes when they first started the yoga for trauma program at the Trauma Justice Center, most of the people dropped out (van der Kolk, 2015). The reason? It was too complicated. They greatly simplified the yoga practice and people stayed. 'More is not better, more is confusing'.

**The Puzzle Pieces – Choosing Poses:** To review, a quick way to assess if a pose is trauma-informed is one key question: what is the perceived level of vulnerability? Or, quite simply, where are the hips? Where is the head? Can someone open their eyes and immediately assess the room? These are factors in someone's perceived sense of safety. Such poses as crescent stretches, warriors one and two, tree pose, and kneeling lunges meet the trauma-informed visual test.

- **Put My Hips Where?** Such poses as a forward fold, child's pose, downward dog, or happy baby all present as vulnerable body postures. A teacher offered at the end of a workshop that now he understood why the women in his free community class refused to do child's pose. He had thought they were simply being difficult. He is a physically large male. These women were immigrants and refugees. He said, "I hadn't even considered any of these points. Now I get it. Boy, now I get it." But not so fast.
- **Who's in Charge?** However, these considerations do not mean certain poses are never taught. Instead, vulnerable poses are something toward which to move, done as someone feels more in control of their bodies and better able to manage their physiological responses. Feeling safe in your body after choosing to lie in happy baby, with soles of the feet together and inner thighs exposed, can be empowering.

One day a woman with a military sexual trauma diagnosis, knowing she and I were alone and the door was locked from the inside, set herself up in this way. She lay back over one bolster and used two to support her knees. With her heels together and her thighs open, she put a blanket over her legs. I assume she felt today was the day to try something new and empowering, as it was not my suggestion. Another woman with a trauma history told me she was really loving a new aerial yoga class. Clearly, she felt in control of herself.

**The Deep End of the Pool:** To avoid tossing people into the deep end of the pool, how could a more vulnerable pose be added? Test the waters in a small class comfortable with you, with the space, and with others in the group.

**You First:** Again, before you suggest changing locations, be confident everyone would be comfortable with what is in fact a disruption. For the 'Final Stretch' (p. 167), after several months, you might demonstrate a legs-up-the-wall pose, with any props that already are part of your practice. Someone can try it today if they like but normalize not wanting to try it with 'different days, different stretches'. I have had classes with no takers, and classes in which people happily set themselves up with props and a sprig of herb under their noses (not my suggestion). Maybe after a few weeks, the legs-up-the-wall options can include the soles of the feet together or bending the knees with feet on the wall. Adding the cue, "You are never stuck, you can always change how you have arranged yourself," continues to build a sense of safety. 'Teach to Empower'.

## To Close: Ways to End Strong

Yoga developed as a way to use breathwork and movement to create ease in still-ness. Or quite literally, to get the wiggles out. A period of stillness and quiet may be difficult or even agitating for anyone, yet even more challenging for someone who has experienced trauma. However, you can incorporate techniques to sup-port trauma recovery and to build resiliency skills. In a 60-to-90-minute prac-tice, I suggest leaving 15 minutes for the 'Final Stretch' sequence.

As you might expect, ending the class is so much more than quiet. There are many suggestions in this section. You can start small and add ideas as you like. Including 'Get Yourself Set Up' to 'Social Connection' takes 15 minutes. These ideas take longer to read about than to do. The simple script for the 'Final Stretch' as well as the suggested steps, are available as an audio (MP3) and as a script to download and add to your clipboard notes (Appendix C: Supplemental Resources).

A side note on how I developed 'Final Stretch' may help you adapt it for your personal or professional needs. To avoid the possible trigger word *relax*, I set-tled on calling it 'Final Stretch'. You may come up with another phrase, but calling it relaxation or corpse pose is potentially triggering. Then using 'your voice is a thread to safety' as a guide, I created a body-based meditation using simple breathwork and gentle movements.

A veteran told me a class ending in ten minutes of total silence with noth-ing to do had created such agitation that she started to cry and had to leave. With no 'voice as a thread to safety' and no body-based grounding guidance, there were many missed opportunities to end strong. Let's look at some steps to create that strong ending.

1. **'Get Yourself Set Up':** Some classes do not have mats, lying down is not appropriate, or being on the floor may not feel safe. Fortunately, yoga is flexible. The 'Final Stretch' easily can be done seated (chair or floor). People tell me that the phrase 'get yourself set up' makes them feel in control.

   **You Set the Stage.** "Lie down, close your eyes, and follow along as I guide you through a progressive relaxation." What does that mean? And where does it end up? Those well-intended words can seem directive, triggering, and distracting. There is no time boundary, no options for how to arrange one-self, and no clear, specific explanation of what will be happening. A clinician shared with me, "I remember the first time I did savasana (final relaxation) in a class I was concerned about how I would know that it was time to sit up. I had no idea that the teacher cued it. It kept me tense." I remember similar experiences.

To maintain that flowin' feeling as you segue to what some consider the peak pose of any practice, you can say after your last pose: "If you like, as YOU breathe in, gently close your fingers or make a fist ... As YOU breathe out, release the fingers. That is tensing and releasing to consciously reduce muscle tension. For the last part of our practice, you can follow along if you like as I guide this tense and release practice in our 'Final Stretch'. When you are ready, you can get yourself set up for 'Final Stretch'."

**Avoid the Mad Dash.** You have worked to maintain a predictable room, which includes everyone staying on their mats or by their chairs. To avoid a mad dash for more props, plan so everyone already has what they need at the start of class. A simple offer keeps the calm. "Okay, I can bring anyone another blanket or mat if you like." Everyone knows why you are moving around the room. Again (and again), it is important to keep talk-ing as someone may already be lying down with their eyes closed. "I am bringing Cindy an extra mat. Now I am walking back to my mat." It may seem silly, but it is not. It maintains predictability. Someone may think or *feel*, "Anytime Yael leaves her mat, she is talking, so I always know where she is in the room. I can close my eyes, no surprises."

**It's a Setup.** "You have options to get yourself set up. You can be seated, or you may like to lie down today, using your blanket or extra mat." This time is the only point at which I demonstrate the choices as I keep talk-ing about what I am demonstrating: perhaps a rolled-up mat under the knees, perhaps lying over a bolster or rolled-up blanket. But again, your voice is the play-by-play, as some people will already be lying down, eyes closed. Include, "You may want to try something *new* today and notice if it feels like a comfortable place to start. Remember, you can always change how you set yourself up. You are never stuck."

2. **Making Sense:** We always come back to the senses because it is how we gather information to make sense of our world. A trauma-informed approach uses various grounding options for ending strong.

   **Smell and Touch.** Please review the science section on why strong scents in your space can be potent triggers (p. 15). Offering a fresh herb (not essences) avoids introducing intrusive or triggering smells. I have these mystery mints in my garden: apple, chocolate, pineapple, spearmint, peppermint, lemon balm, and catmint. At the end, people share guesses on today's mint. I also have herbs with leaves that are soft, feathery, waxy, smooth, and delicate. Now let's add another sense.

**Hearing.** 'Your voice is a thread to safety' is a key. "As you get yourselves set up, I am going to walk around the inside of *our* circle (reinforce a sense of community). Today I have a mystery mint from my garden." To avoid possible triggers, I identify it as a mint or name today's herb. "I also have stones from the Maine rocky coast. So, I as I walk around, you can choose something to hold if you like. Perhaps you'd like one in each hand." You can see why using 'your voice as the thread to safety' is not a small point. Imagine how someone walking quietly around the room, not talking, could be quite stressful. On a similar note, give verbal notice before introducing a new sound: "Now I am going to ring the singing bowl three times."

**One More Sense – Social Connection.** Sharing is an opportunity to express yourself. What do I offer? I share shells, rocks, pressed leaves/ferns, pinecones, and a variety of herbs with many textures and smells. You may have noted I say where I collected them. There is the option for someone to keep the offerings. Some return from trips and bring shells or rocks to add to our centerpiece collection. Did you note the two healing components in trauma recovery? Building community and thinking about the future. Some people save a shell or a piece of pressed fern to put at the front of their mats every class. Someone told me she put the rock from southern Utah in her collection by her bed, and she told me what other rocks she had. Points of connection.

3.  **'Final Stretch' – A Guided, Body-based Meditation:** Again, this section looks like a lot, but after the 'Final Stretch' script, much of the text is explanations for you. As you read the script, you can see it uses an easy-to-remember, fill-in-the-blank from fingers to toes format. It's why years later, a veteran texted me to say that the first ten minutes of her physical therapy was heat and electricity. "I have discovered that your 'Final Stretch' is perfect for that time."

## 'Final Stretch' Script

"In 'Final Stretch' we practice tightening muscles and then releasing them. Only tighten your muscles in a comfortable way. If you like, on YOUR next breath in, close the fingers on one hand. As YOU breathe out, release. The suggestion is to take long, slow breaths out that *can* lower heart rate, lower blood pressure, and lower muscle tension. Now if you like, on YOUR next breath in, close the fingers on the other hand. On YOUR breath out, release. Even small movements or visualizing the movements have benefits. Eyes open or eyes closed, your choice. I keep my eyes open so I can let you know if someone joins us. We always do both sides. I start on the left. Again, follow along if you like."

I.  **Tense/Release Hands to Feet**

"As YOU breathe in, close the *fingers* on your left hand … As YOU breathe out, release.

As YOU breathe in, close the *fingers* and tighten your *forearm* … As YOU breathe out, release. Always move and breathe in a comfortable way.

On YOUR next breath in, tighten your *shoulder* … As YOU breathe out, release.

As YOU breathe in, tighten the left side of your *back*, as YOU breathe out, release.

As YOU breathe in, tighten the muscles around your left *hip* … As YOU breathe out, release.

On YOUR next breath in, press down on your left *heel* … As YOU breathe out, release."

II.  **Tense/Release Each Side**

"Now keep breathing as you tighten every muscle you would like on your left side …

Perhaps your fist … forearm … shoulder … jaw … back … hip … leg. (*Say slowly.*)

When the muscles are as tight as YOU would like them to be *today*, use YOUR next breath out to release …

Perhaps your fist … forearm … shoulder … jaw … back … hip … leg. (*Say slowly.*)

Notice YOUR next breath in, chest and belly lift …

As YOU breathe out, feel your left side fully supported.

Notice YOUR next breath in, chest and belly lift …

As YOU breathe out, feel your left side get heavy.

Before we do the other side, make any adjustments so you are comfortable for the next few minutes … you are never stuck." (*Repeat I. and II. slowly on the other side. Then go to III.*)

People tell me they had no idea they clenched their jaws until we did "that jaw thing."

### III.   'Feel the Breath'/'Take Up Space'/Comfortable Seat

1) **'Feel the Breath':** "If you like, put one or both hands over your heart … put one or both hands over your heart. Let's practice 5 breaths. Feel the breath in … Feel the breath out. (*Say 2 times slowly.*) Now if you like, say the next 3 to yourself in your mind, because *you* are always with you. (*Say slowly during this time to avoid dead air*: "Don't rush your words … Don't rush your breath … Take your time with your words … Take your time with your breath.)

2) **'Take Up Space'** "When you are ready, begin to put more effort into your breath in, if that is comfortable for you today. A longer breath in *can* be energizing. If you like, extend your arms overhead, hands on the floor behind you. 'Take Up Space' as you stretch your fingers wide, stretch your toes … and practice longer breaths in if that is comfortable today. When you are ready, gently bend your knees and roll onto your *right* side, in the interest of personal space so you are facing away from each other."

3) **Comfortable Seat with 'Finger Stretch Breath':** "When you are ready, with your eyes still closed if you like, find a comfortable seat. If you like, gently press one shoulder back … Then press the other shoulder back. Let's practice 3 breaths. As you breathe in, fingers stretch … as you breathe out, release the stretch." (*Say 3 times slowly.*)

### IV.   To End Strong (5 minutes) – Noticing to Social Connection:

Consider: 1) Noticing, 2) 'Make a Plan', 3) A Mindful Moment/*Namaste*, 4) Giving Voice, and 5) Social Connection.

1) **Noticing:** (20 seconds) "Before you open your eyes, notice if you feel better than you did an hour ago. Perhaps notice if you met your intention for your practice, the reason that you came today. Were you able to make it happen for yourself ?" I encourage taking ownership. Blaming someone else is not practicing a helpful life strategy. Your teaching intention was to create a class to practice self-regulation and resiliency skills, so that seemingly simple question gets to the heart of what just happened in the last hour.

2)  **'Make a Plan':** (one minute) I notice that it helps me a lot physically and mentally since I am going through a lot of stress, kids, job, school. You can do yoga anywhere, the thought I used to have about yoga, now I know you can have it anyplace, you don't need a real quiet place. It's given me time to remind myself about myself, so I communicate with myself and most importantly, I do healthy breathing. ~ refugee mother from Sudan

Some people are not aware that simple stretching and breathing breaks can be incorporated throughout their days. One veteran shared, "Wow, I didn't realize I could do this at home!" A teacher shared that someone said, "I haven't done yoga before. I really liked that! I liked the real-life application of doing it in a chair." She then asked if she could utilize (her word) tree pose on her own throughout the day as she needed. 'Teach to Empower'.

The importance of making a plan builds on Dr. Jack Kornfield's idea from his book, *The Wise Heart*. Instead of being captive to pain or stress, recognize the feeling and approach it with a tool. "Oh, this is me feeling stressed" (Kornfield, 2008). It is nothing short of empowering to end every practice with an option to create a two-minute plan that works in real-time. Steps 1, 2, and 3 provide the quick version. Some days you may want to include more.

**Step 1:** "Before you open your eyes, the suggestion is to make a two-minute plan, something you can do later in the day or the night when you want to change how you are feeling."

The following is included to explain to you the reasoning behind this simple suggestion, again *not* for you to explain to someone. "Oh, I know what to do!" can become someone's first response. With a bit of practice, it can become a habit: that is, the brain rewires as someone uses alternate pathways for more adaptive responses. I started using the phrase, "when you want to change how you are feeling" because it is nondirective, empowering, and open-ended. Someone may be feeling collapsed and sad. Or someone may be feeling anxious or agitated. I encourage you to find empowering phrases that resonate with you."

**Step 2:** "If you like, pick one breath that we did today – we did 'The Wave Breath', 'Feel the Breath', and the 'Anytime, Anywhere Breath'. Remember, choosing how you breathe is a way to manage how you feel. It's body physiology."

**Step 3:** "Now, if you like, add one stretch you might want to do later. Maybe it was shoulder rolls or crescent stretch. (Give 2 suggestions so no one feels adrift.) You now have a 2-minute plan, a 5-part breath, and a simple stretch to do later when you want to change how you are feeling."

**Variations:** 'Make a Plan' can extend to include someone doing (or visualizing themselves doing) the breathwork and then the stretch for somatic reinforcement. A general cue: "As YOU breathe in, hands move ... As YOU breathe out, release. (*Say 5 times slowly.*) I might say, "Notice if you had an opportunity this past week to use a breathing break to change how you're feeling. If you did, you were able to practice interrupting your body's stress cycle. And if you didn't, that's good news too. You have something easy to try this week." It's judgement free. Most of us respond well to positivity.

3) **A Mindful Moment/Namaste:** (20 seconds) "We can end a yoga practice by putting our palms together (**Variation**). We can say a word that means, loosely translated, the goodness or kindness in me recognizes the goodness or kindness in you. That word is namaste. If you like, to each other and especially to yourself, we can say, namaste." I have had the most unlikely people share that "especially to yourself" held special meaning for them. For some, it gave them the awareness to be more assertive or to practice more self-care. 'Seeds planted'. Namaste is the only Sanskrit word I use in a trauma-informed class, and the only time palms are together. **Variation:** Never wanting to miss a grounding opportunity, when palms press together, "Notice if your palms feel warm today," or "Gently press your palms together ... Then release the press," or "Press your palms together as firmly as comfortable ... Then press them so they are gently touching."

4) **Giving Voice:** (#4 and #5 together take 4 minutes) In trauma recovery, being heard or practicing self-expression can be an empowering step. Again, it must be stressed that giving voice pertains *only* to the yoga practice *not* to someone's trauma. As always, different groups, different approaches. I will share some techniques to consider as you develop and iterate your programs.

**Do You Have Aquamarine?** After we say namaste, I walk around the inside of our circle and offer an optional evaluation form, a choice of colored pens, and a baked good. It is interesting how many pause to choose a specific color. Create any opportunity to practice making choices, an action that empowers. I learn what is working and what can be improved. People write extra information. A transgender person added a line under the "Reasons I Came to Yoga: Stay out of Hospital (psych unit)" and then checked it. A retired military nurse with both PTSD and military sexual trauma diagnoses told me writing for these few moments after class gave her time to think about what she had gotten out of today's class. To her, it was a valuable exercise as otherwise she would not have taken the time. Another written response to "What did you enjoy about yoga today?" was "Being able to settle into some depth of my emotions – while at the same time not letting them overwhelm me." Giving voice. Sample forms to use as a template are found Appendix C: Supplemental Resources. Then make it your own.

5) **Social Connection:** For years I baked for my classes. Having raised three boys, I still can't go anywhere without food to share. Another veteran, a retired nurse practitioner and a German refugee in WW2 started bringing amazing baked goods to share. I baked, but she was an artist, sparing no expense with time or ingredients. The groups gave her much deserved praise and thanks. She started including recipes with her offerings. She made these social connections for two years, until our classes were remote. She continued to share her virtual treats, photographs, and recipes included.

**It's a Circle Thing:** With a small group I know well, sometimes before we say namaste I will say, "Let's go around the circle, and if you like, share one thing you noticed about the practice today. Or simply look to the next person. So, 'I noticed that ...'" So far, no one has opted out of sharing. Of course, you will have a sense of how worthwhile the exercise is for your group. Occasionally, I will say, "Let's go around the circle, and if you like, share one small thing for which you are grateful today." Thank you, James Fox of the Prison Yoga Project for chatting with me about the benefits of such an exercise. In a larger group, it may be more appropriate to say, "Perhaps give yourself a few moments to notice to yourself something about your practice today." If suggesting people notice to themselves, doing it before you say namaste avoids the bustle of class ending.

For some groups, written expression is not the first choice. With refugees, I will pass my phone around to record responses. They repeat the prompt I give to each person: "Today I noticed that ..." The positive and heart-felt responses inspire me. In one class, someone translated the prompt, and the person recorded their answer in their language. Asking veterans is heartening as well. You don't ask, you don't know. I included those joining through telehealth by holding my phone to the screen. You can hear some of these comments, including the Sudanese mother's quote in the 'make a plan' section, at this link: www.greentreeyoga.org/noticed. As you get to know your groups, you can find ways to build connections. You can find ways to help someone master yoga, in the way that T.K.V. Desikachar defined mastery: "Mastery of Yoga is really measured by how it influences our day-to-day living, how it enhances our relationships, how it promotes clarity and peace of mind" (Desikachar, 1999).

**Staying After for Extra Help:** Someone may ask about ideas for back pain. After I explain they should check with their medical providers, I mention some benefits as I teach my class as planned. I add that after class, I will offer more suggestions on back stretches to those interested. One suggestion is child's pose (big toes touching, knees apart), with someone standing over you with hands spaced apart on your back. One hand (fingers facing toward the head) presses toward the head and one hand (fingers facing back) presses back. "Eeek," you may be thinking, and rightly so. But I am the one in the child's pose, and I talk someone through my suggestions. Then I ask if anyone would like to try it. There may be some heart-warming interactions as people pair to help each other. Social support strengthened, connections made, and windows of tolerance widened.

Another back stretch suggestion is to get set up in 'Kitchen Stretch' (p. 237), a half forward fold with palms on the wall or back of a chair. Again, I am the person in the position with my hips pressed back. Again, I talk someone through the adjustment, which is to stand behind me and press the heels of their hands down and back from the top of the hip bone. Some say they will try it at home, while others want to try it with a partner or with me. Please note, these are not suggestions I would ever make *during* a class. Yet if someone opts to learn new things after class, it is empowering, builds social connection, and can help manage neck and back pain.

## Activities to Compliment Your Practice

The following activities were developed to follow the Warrior Renew program at the Salt Lake City Veterans Administration (VA) (Katz, 2014). Lori Katz, PhD, offers this information on her program. The Warrior Renew program is designed to treat the most salient issues for those who have experienced sexual trauma and abuse manifesting as disrupted sleep, anger, self-blame, and grief. It also addresses such interpersonal factors as examining relationship patterns, and perceptions of self in relationships. It is delivered in a group to build trust, community, and communication skills. It incorporates cognitive (mind) and experiential (body) strategies for healing. Such activities as yoga and creative self-expression through art are well-suited to augment this approach as they support integrating Warrior Renew material through cognitive-experiential modalities. More specifically, yoga helps dislodge physical and emotional constriction, while supporting people to open, expand, and breathe. This supports Warrior Renew skills for emotion regulation. Art helps with symbolic expression (L.J. Katz, personal communication, May 26, 2023).

## Journaling

When I decided to include 30 minutes of journaling, I looked for a template. None met my intentions, so I developed my own. I did not want gaping blank pages to cause stress, so I offered structured options: written prompts, colorful pens, quotes, and a variety of art materials. A few words on the colorful pens. One woman kept saying, "I want the green one. Yes, I want the green one." She would pause and repeat. I thought it was odd, as I was not denying anyone pens, until she laughed and said, "We practiced making little choices today in group." I knew I was on the right track with colored pens. Many ideas on prompts and quotes that can serve as seed crystals for journaling are available (Appendix C: Supplemental Resources). I will note that people were eager to use all the resources offered. 'Small choices. Small points of awareness. Small movements toward trauma recovery'.

Veterans would come each week during the eight-week Warrior Renew program. Some arrived seeming dazed and confused. I could see visible changes in their demeanors during the yoga hour. Our yoga circle would transform as we shared tea and baked goods and wrote in personal journals. The following comments from various program cohorts can give you a sense of how you can expand the benefits of your yoga class.

One veteran glued a photo of her three-year-old self on her journal cover, saying that was the last time she remembered not feeling trauma. She was 63 years old. Another told us she had to leave early to get back to Valor House (veteran housing) about a debriefing: a 24-year-old resident had committed suicide by cop. She asked if it were okay if she journaled before she left, she really wanted to do that first. Another woman commented that the feathers she glued on the journal cover were like a soft place to land. Someone else wrapped colorful yarns around her cover, saying, "Maybe after this, I won't feel all bound up." When someone arrived at a different yoga class I offered, she asked, "Can I just do my journal now, if that's okay, I just came from my therapist." Sitting in a quiet corner to journal seemed part of her processing. One day a veteran did ten minutes of yoga, then asked for her journal and journal prompts to take home. She said she was so scattered because she'd taken on everyone's things in group. She used words from our class: "I just need to give myself a moment …" This phrase, from David Emerson is one I use in class. To me it always sounds like a gift.

At the Warrior Renew graduation ceremony, one veteran held up her favorite journal entry prompt, a lotus picture and Buddhist quote, "May you be like the lotus, at home in the muddy water." She had written in her journal and now read to us: "This is now I now feel: rooted and able to move in the muddy water, and yet there is a flower blooming on top." I had the opportunity to meet several of the women a year or two after our class, and they each said how rereading their journals had been very powerful – to see where they were then and where they were now. Another woman wrote me that the class was "a wonderful opportunity to process feelings by writing endlessly … over tea and sweets and all that female camaraderie."

## Art Projects

After people journaled for 30 minutes, we would work on some craft for another 30 minutes: decorating a cap or a tote bag. Each week for eight weeks I would bring in something new to add. Pompoms, foam stickers, glitter glue, fancy yarns, and textured felt are some examples. It also kept me actively engaged as exploring craft stores was new to me. As one astute person told our group, "You know, this is really art therapy. It's great. I haven't done things like this since I was a kid."

One woman shared after doing the craft and journal entry, "I feel so loved. You know, I have never felt loved." On the cap project: "It was like a blank slate. I didn't know what you would bring and what you wanted us to do. Now I look forward to it." Someone glued pompoms on her cap and said, "This is for the little girl I once was and the woman I now am who saved her." Another said the cap "is like a canvas … I can write my story." Someone else looked at them in our group circle: "Did you notice the caps get bolder every week?" One cohort decorated SOLA STIKK®, information that is available for free on the GreenTREE Yoga website. The many possibilities can only stoke the imagination.

**\*\*\*\*\*\*\*\*\***

**To Recap:** Giving yourself the time to consider why simple breathwork and movement can be key in trauma recovery and building resiliency skills has brought you here. You are set up to make a plan. A strong class plan accounts for time (too much, too little), keeping the flow, differing abilities, and the simple breathwork and movement practices. A yoga practice has a beginning, a middle, and an end, designed to use the breath, the body, and the mind to reset the nervous system. You can make each part trauma-informed using the guide of building a sense of safety, supporting empowerment, and maintaining simplicity. There are many activities to complement any yoga practice, including art and journaling. Chapter 11 provides descriptions, outlines, and scripts for all the practice sequences.

## References

Calhoun, Yael. (2025). *Art and Yoga for Children with Differing Needs and Autism: Improve Body Awareness, Sensory Integration, and Emotional Regulation.* London: Singing Dragon Press.

Desikachar, T. K. V. (1999). *The Heart of Yoga.* Rochester, VT: Inner Traditions.

Doidge, Norman. (2016). *The Brain's Way of Healing: Remarkable Discoveries and Recoveries from the Frontiers of Neuroplasticity.* New York: Penguin Life, p. 166.

Katz, Lori. (2014). *Warrior Renew: Healing from Military Sexual Trauma.* New York: Springer Press.

Kornfield, Jack. (2008). *The Wise Heart.* New York: Bantom Books.

Van der Kolk, Bessel A. (2015). *The Body Keeps the Score: Brain, Mind, and Body in the Healing of Trauma.* New York: Penguin Books.

## 10

# Immigrant/Refugee/ ESOL Populations

This chapter builds on previous ones while considering the unique needs of refugees, immigrants, and English as a second or other language (ESOL) groups. Chapter 11's practice sequence V ('All Together Now', p. 220) is specifically for refugee and immigrant groups. Should you have an opportunity to teach these groups, there are many ways to make what you offer more accessible. Be confident that preparing with awareness and clear intentions will greatly improve your overall teaching skills. You may have first-hand experience teaching these groups, but it can still be worthwhile to run through these ideas.

A sense of safety remains paramount, possibly even more so in groups with complex traumas and major life disruptions. Often people come from unsafe homes and countries. English is not their first language, contributing to their sense of isolation. They may not have found new, meaningful work or had the opportunity to reconnect to a community. Much of the new culture may seem strange and stressful.

You may teach one class, or you may have the opportunity to teach a series of classes and develop personal connections. Your first teaching consideration is to identify your trauma-informed tools to help rebuild a sense of safety. Let's make a list. You will see some overlap from previous trauma-informed protocols. But not surprisingly, there are new considerations for this unique population. Teaching refugees and immigrants is a special opportunity for you to practice 'Trust the Yoga' and 'Show, Don't Tell'.

## Building Safety

### You Are the Message: 'Your Voice Is a Thread to Safety'

Perhaps the most important thing you bring to class is yourself. The groups may speak little or no English. First, a note on teaching with an interpreter.

DOI: 10.4324/9781003308836-13

A good interpreter will speak almost with you, so there is no break in the flow. People listen to the interpreter, but they keep attuned to your face, voice, movements, and breath. If you do not have an interpreter, you may feel at a teaching disadvantage. However, another key dimension to language is the prosody (rhythm and intonations) of your voice. How you say words, not the words themselves, and your facial expressions can effectively convey a sense of safety

I experienced 'my voice is a thread to safety' as I taught a one-time class after a women's sewing skills group. Many languages were spoken, none of which was English. Not only was the group new to me, but I had never taught non-English speakers without an interpreter. However, I heard my friend's voice in my mind. He had worked with refugees for years, and I heard him say, "Just teach, they will follow you. I am reminding you what I have learned from you." Thank you, Cameron! Buoyed by these words, I pressed on. I used my regular teaching cues because that guided *me*. Using familiar words and phrases kept my voice and facial expressions calm, signaling we are safe here. I noticed they followed my every movement and my breathing. I followed their cues of smiles and nods and gentle movements. Success. I can imagine the questions they were asking themselves or processing on some subcortical level: "Do I want to do what she is doing? Are we still safe in this room? Do I want to feel as she is feeling, based on her facial expressions and voice?" My suggestion is not to overthink what you are saying. Rely on your familiar trauma-informed protocols. But above all, 'Trust the Yoga'.

## Let Me Count the Ways

The guiding idea is simple: maximize any opportunity to create connections. You can incorporate and adapt in ways that serve your intentions, resources, and personality.

**The Room:** Given the high degrees of pain and of physical and emotional trauma in these groups, I arrange chairs in a circle with ample room on each side. Yoga mats are not necessary and may cause stress from being something new. Be confident chairs in a circle or semicircle can create a lovely practice. People like to help set up the room, not surprising since moving and directed action can reduce stress. I always bring food and flowers or some centerpiece for our circle. One program coordinator told me that she could not believe the change in the demeanor of the group, just finishing an ESOL class, when I quietly came in and put the healthy snacks, the flowers, and the herbs on the back table. To me, the offerings are a small way to build a sense of trust, safety, and stability in our group.

**'Opening Connections' – Plan on It: (10 minutes)** This piece of the practice is not extra. In my experience, it is key to activating the social engagement system. Please factor in the time on your clipboard schedule: 'Opening Connections' (10 minutes). For an hour class, I have a place with healthy food arranged on a side table and the name cards (folded index cards) ready to put on the floor in front of each chair.

- **Let's Eat!** I offer the food first. We know that eating together activates the social engagement system. We sit in our chair circle and eat the offerings of healthy snacks – fruits, baked goods, and nuts. It is important to note that some people arrive hungry, as they may not have extra food at home or didn't eat before rushing their kids to school. A note on the food: I always bring extra. Women gratefully accepted it, many saying it was for their kids after school. I remember one woman held out a full plate and asked, "Are you sure you don't need it?"
- **All in a Name.** Social connection plays center stage with these groups. They are away from their familiar points of connection: people, places, and things. Again, in front of each of us on the floor is a small folded index card with our names. We go around the circle and introduce ourselves. My attempts to say their beautiful names always led to some smiles as I often did not succeed. We welcome those new to the group, for some may have just arrived in this new country. One woman came to our class the day after she had arrived from Albania. Some may share what yoga break they did at home last week or taught to a friend. I walk around the inside of the circle and offer sprigs of this week's herb. Someone usually has a comment on what it is called at home or how they use it.

It surprised me one week someone who had been quite negative during class returned to thank me for the nice food – point of connection. Another time, someone had to leave during class for legal asylum guidance. She returned to tell me, without much English, how the breathing (she did the hand movements) helped her so much.

- **Word of the Day.** Choose a word relevant to the day's practice: for example, strong, breathe, or calm. Ask people to share the word in their language. Perhaps write the words on a board (usually handy after an ESOL class). Passing your phone around so people can say the word in their language sets you up to make a chart for the next week as a fun review.

I struggle with languages, so it was a nice connection as people patiently tried to teach me to count in Arabic, Urdu, Swahili, and Farsi. And again, some people find a shared language with people from other countries, as it is not uncommon for refugees to speak more than one language – some speak many.

**Ready to Go.** Plates are cleared. We begin our practice, already having connected for 10 minutes through food, introductions, sharing languages, and cooking stories.

## Boundaries

There are two types of interactions: ones that support your efforts to build community and safety and ones that do not. You want to encourage group interactions to support someone feeling heard and seen. So, your task is to balance group connections with the class flow. Your task is to balance group connections with the quiet needed for someone to connect with their breath and their bodily sensations. With awareness and effort, you can find your own rhythm. Clear and respectful boundaries become an important management tool.

**'Silly Shake and Stretch':** People may engage in nervous laughter or tell others what to do. I was told in the refugee camps, this behavior was common. In addition, someone new to the group may feel anxious. After 'Opening Connections', one way to manage nervous behavior is the two-minute 'Silly Shake and Stretch' as discussed in Chapter 11 (220). Inspired by the work of Peter Levine, PhD, and James Gordon, MD, I named and tried it in all female groups (Levine, 1997; Gordon, 2019/2021). It is popular – a lot of silly moving and shaking, followed by 'Feel the Breath' (p. 125). You may find you're now looking at a different group. However, be sensitive to the fact that for some, shaking creates an out-of-control feeling or simply hurts. It is good practice to offer the option of gently moving and stretching first, then offer the shaking and being silly. Later, another round of 'Silly Shake and Stretch' can embrace the laughing, contain it, and allow you to move on. The importance of bringing a sense of play (lila) to trauma recovery is discussed on pages 24/144.

**The Direct Approach:** Disruptive chatter or negative comments can be distracting. It can be effective to say, "Okay, let's use this time to do some yoga. We can chat after class." If language is an issue, putting your finger to your mouth in the "shhh" sign can work. Again, someone may be nervous or not know what is expected. You might even ask someone for the please be quiet phrase in their language to bring some levity to the situation. As the teacher, feel confident that you are being respectful of everyone's time and need for safety by keeping clear boundaries.

**It's the Little Ones:** Some facilities have childcare, so the adults can focus on themselves for an hour. But children often appear, which can create stress for the parents if they are trying to keep the children quiet. The boundary I have found most useful is to include the children in the practice. A two-year-old pulling apart the flowers in the center of our circle? Smile and carry on. The message is positive: one does not need to be alone or have total quiet to do yoga. You have created a welcoming space. You stay calm. These safety cues come across in your voice and facial expression. A teacher who was observing my class later wrote, "I liked how you allowed the children to flow in and out and touch things and highlighted them moving with us. The atmosphere felt light, safe and happy." Thank you, Amy! One day I was about to start 'Opening Connections', and I looked at a mom with her two-year-old perched on her lap. At the sound of my voice, the two-year-old started doing 'The Wave Breath' hand gestures from the previous week.

**Cultural Respect:** Cultural awareness is part of the boundary of safety. Your dress and your speech are perhaps the most obvious demonstration of cultural respect. If you have demonstrated your respect by modest dress and speech, and you do something culturally inappropriate, as happened to me with a suggestion about a foot stretch in a Muslim group, someone will nicely and without taking offense, say, "Oh, we can't do that." In one community leader training I did, women from 15 tribes and countries participated. Be aware that there can be tribal and other cultural tensions within a group. Again, awareness is the first step in addressing any potential issues.

## Social Support in Action

**Connections Made:** Teaching a class series allows you more ways to connect with your group. Perhaps someone texts to let you know they won't be there today. Obviously, carefully observe privacy. You can simply share with the group at 'Opening Connections' that Aisha won't be joining this week, but she will see us next week. You may notice more people keeping in touch. As an example, an older woman missed a few weeks because she had surgery. In a card, I wrote a short sentence in English and invited everyone to write it in their language and sign it. It was quite the card, different languages, different alphabets. Her friend delivered it, and the next week reported how touched the woman had been to be in our thoughts. One week someone texted she was running late so wouldn't come as she didn't want to interrupt. I texted back, "Join when you can, please come!" I told the group, providing predictability. She arrived, bearing handfuls of mint to share and seemed grateful to be welcomed.

**Group Voice:** I had to rework my ideas about talking during class because social connection is so important to trauma recovery and building resiliency skills. As Bessel van der Kolk and Stephen Porges note, social connection is one of the strongest protective factors against trauma and in building resiliency skills (van der Kolk, 2015; Porges, 2017). Encouraging people to interact, within your clear boundaries, can strengthen social connection and serve as additional safety cues. Not only is your voice a safety cue, but a group speaking together can support self-regulation (van der Kolk, 2015; Porges, 2017). The healing power of singing, chanting, and group prayers celebrates that body physiology. In what ways can you use this idea to your teaching advantage? The following suggestions have worked well in my classes.

**Sharing Language, Laughter, and Movement:** Laughter can reduce stress as it creates longer breaths out. Think of a time when you may have laughed much more than a situation warranted. Laughter may be the body's way of reducing stress. Working with children at low-income schools where many languages are spoken, I found that group counting in different languages paired with movement did two things. It created a lovely physical group rhythm and also some opportunities to speak and laugh together.

I easily adapted a warrior one flow for the ESOL groups. Standing in a circle, everyone steps one foot forward 'in a way that feels good or comfortable today'. Ask if someone would like to count in their language. As someone says *one* in Somali, we all raise our arms in peaceful warrior one. Then together, as we release our arms, we say *one* in Somali. After three times, we change sides with another language volunteer. There can be a lovely synchronicity as you all speak, breathe, laugh, and move as a group.

Over the weeks, I would ask how many times we should do one side. Someone would say, "Ten times!" We would all laugh. "It's an option, do what feels good or comfortable today." I noticed when doing something in another language and all speaking together, people wanted to move much more. A bit of fun created opportunities for personal growth, for social connection, and for being heard.

One last note on cueing movement is not to cue alignment. Be sensitive to women in non-yoga clothing. Someone will follow your visual cues as best they can. For warrior one, step one foot back, as in a lunge, as it's much less stress on the hips. Set everyone up for success. Someone can find what they need today without you micromanaging. 'Trust the Yoga'.

**Simply Showing Up – Physical Inclusion:** In a group that met after a sewing skills class, a woman holding a newborn told me she could not join the class today because stretching really hurt. I could feel the group deflate. So, I smiled and invited her to bring her infant and sit in our circle if she liked and simply breathe with us. That was all I said. She rather tentatively joined us, baby in the carrier next to her, and proceeded to do every stretch and breath with our group.

**Sharing Favorites:** Taking a few minutes in the middle of a class to share favorite poses or five-part breaths can provide a way to keep everyone engaged. The way you offer it depends on the group. In some groups, it may be helpful to say you are going to go around the circle, if someone would like to share, great. If not, just keep going. Another way is to ask for volunteers: "Let's have four suggestions." If time allows, I find going around the circle creates a lovely sharing experience. Please note the difference. Someone may not want to draw attention to themselves by volunteering but will gladly share if it's their turn.

## Supporting Empowerment

**Choice:** There may be many chronic pain issues in this population, so it is important to continually offer, "Anything we do standing, we can do seated. Or anything we do seated, you can do standing." In these classes, it is helpful to demonstrate the choice of standing or sitting as you say it, smiling and nodding as you do. Remember, sitting is uncomfortable for some, so practicing making choices continues to build that sense of safety. Support someone finding what they need today by including "the suggestion is …" and "you are never stuck" in cues. Sometimes I ask someone to translate these key points. An older woman in my class spoke Urdu, so her friend translated as I spoke. I was sitting on the other side of her in our circle. She leaned over and kept gently squeezing my hand as she spoke softly to me in Urdu. Her friend told me she was saying, "It means so much to me that you said I can do less, it feels really good to just move a little. Thank you." 'Small choices. Small points of awareness. Small movements toward trauma recovery'.

**Breathwork – Ready to Go:** After several classes, I teach a five-part breathing break with this change as language allows. After three breaths: "Now, if you like, practice 2 more breaths, saying it to yourself in your mind. Because you are always with you." People tell me the phrase 'you are always with you' is helpful.

**Giving Voice:** I came to working with refugees after many years of working with English speakers. In my experience, asking if anyone had something on which they wanted to work often led to oversharing and easily could bring everyone down. However, I was inspired by a clinical social worker friend, who shared how it was a positive experience to inquire as to specific concerns the refugees were experiencing – back, hip, neck. So, after several weeks, once we had a rhythm to the class, I inquired. Several people offered neck and low back, and a chorus of agreement followed. I addressed the concerns as I taught my planned class. I was touched by how grateful people were, expressed with verbal thanks and nods after class. They were not looking to create a gripe session but simply were grateful to be given a voice.

**A Sense of Purpose:** Attending a yoga class or stretching and breathing class, can provide a sense of purpose for someone's day. Many who have experienced trauma "have lost their sense of purpose and direction" (van der Kolk, 2015). A yoga class can provide a bit of direction. "I am going to do yoga now." Or "I want to do yoga now." Support small steps to rebuilding a life in a new country.

**You Be the Teacher:** Another way to add variety to the practice is to invite someone to teach a pose or a breath to the group during favorites. This offer accomplishes several things. It can deepen the sense of community in the group. Teaching also allows someone to experience how it might feel to share the break at home or at work. During 'Opening Connections', asking who taught a yoga break to someone reinforces that yoga is to share. 'Plant seeds'.

**Room for Personal Growth:** Including some of the same poses each week provides consistency. When you say, "Let's set up for tree pose," someone may feel curious about how the pose will feel this week. Someone also may experience a sense of personal growth and personal mastery from one week to the next. It can be fun to have one or two poses with an element of challenge. For example, doing tree pose while standing by a chair allows for many easy-to-understand visual options. Often people like feeling their muscles working, a way to reconnect with their bodies. One Iraqi refugee shared, "I am with my body now, before I was not with my body."

**Support Materials:** Sharing a one page handout of a breathwork and simple pose you practiced today empowers someone to practice at home or at work. Sharing an MP3 or MP4 of that *one* break also can be helpful. Appendix C: Supplemental Resources has specific links to share one break at a time. Remember, 'More is not better, more is confusing'.

## Maintaining Simplicity

It seems obvious but still worth a quick review. Simplicity is the key. In addition to unresolved trauma limiting verbal processing, there are language considerations as well. So, keeping your cues simple, specific, and body-based is important. Keeping the words and phrases consistent is key. To cue, "Lift your arm toward the ceiling" on one side and "Raise your hand as high as you can" on the other side is not clear. It can be fun to incorporate words the group is learning into your cues. One day the ESOL class was learning body parts already written on the white board behind me, so I made sure to emphasize fingers, toes, hands, feet, legs, and shoulders in my cues.

And, more so than with any group, 'Trust the Yoga' can give *you* confidence. Again, if you think the words are not being understood, keep your flow of your usual trauma-informed cues, keep your rhythm of speech, and 'Trust the Yoga'. And of course, 'Show, Don't Tell'. A refugee or immigrant class is not the place to muse about unrelated topics.

**********

**To Recap:** The most obvious challenge in working with refugees and immigrants may appear to be language. But rebuilding a sense of safety and social connection are the more important challenges. There are many ways to meet these challenges with what you have: your voice, your facial expressions, healthy snacks, sharing languages, creating safe boundaries, building a sense of group, and reciprocity of inclusive banter. My advice is to 'Trust the Yoga' and to have fun creating new connections.

## References

Gordon, James. (2019/2021). *The Transformation: Discovering Wholeness and Healing After Trauma.* New York: Harper One.

Levine, Peter. (1997). *Waking the Tiger: Healing Trauma.* Berkeley: North Atlantic Books, pp. 97–98.

Porges, Stephen. (2017). *The Pocket Guide to the Polyvagal Theory: The Transformative Power of Feeling Safe.* W.W. Norton & Company, pp. 108–109.

Van der Kolk, Bessel A. (2015). *The Body Keeps the Score: Brain, Mind, and Body in the Healing of Trauma.* New York: Penguin Publishing, pp. 79; 166–167.

## 11
# Trauma-informed Phrases and Practice Sequences/Photos

## Practice Sequences: Descriptions and Outlines

The breathwork and yoga poses in these practice sequences are found in all GreenTREE Yoga® trainings, manuals, books, and audio/video recordings. This book's practice sequences are designed specifically for trauma recovery and building resiliency skills. These practices were developed over many years of teaching diverse groups, making the practices a strong starting point from which to develop your programs.

**Format:** To support a variety of teaching opportunities, yoga practices include two formats.

1) Two-to-five-minute breaks: Supplemental resources include teacher scripts. In addition, MP3s (audio), MP4s (video), and handouts can be used as teaching tools and to share with students, clients, and patients.
2) Full practices (30/60/90 minutes): Supplemental resources include the scripts from this chapter to download.

DOI: 10.4324/9781003308836-14

**Photographs:** For easy reference, practice sequence photographs of poses are grouped to show different options and variations. Referring to the photographs can support sharing trauma-informed yoga in ways to meet someone where they are (pp. 228–242).

**The 'Final Stretch':** Practice sequence IV includes the 'Final Stretch' (p. 167), which also is downloadable for easy reference in your clipboard notes. You also can use it to extend any 30-minute practice or incorporate parts to meet your changing program needs. The 'Final Stretch' is not included in the practice sequence for refugees and immigrants for two reasons: 1) floorwork usually is not a good fit; and 2) language considerations can be limiting.

**Breathwork Information and Variations:** Breathwork is a key part of any practice. The suggestion is to give yourself a few moments to review the ideas on sharing breathwork facts on page 125. This chapter's breathwork includes page references from Chapter 7 for background and variations.

**Clipboard Notes:** The suggestion is to download the clipboard notes. You can plan the day's trauma-informed phrases and then use the notes as a guide while you teach. Multiple reasons that a clipboard can be a strong trauma-informed teaching tool are on page 157.

## Phrases to Empower, to Build Body Awareness, and to Build Breath Awareness

These trauma-informed phrases can be included in any practice sequence. Ideas on how you can practice your trauma-informed teaching are in Chapter 5 (p. 101).

**Table 11.1** Phrases to Empower

| Trauma-informed Phrase | When/Why to Use |
|---|---|
| "Anything that we do standing, you can do seated or even lying down. You can always find ways to breathe and move with me." | This phrase says you have no expectations and support someone 'finding a comfortable way to move today'.<br>Offering this option lets everyone know they can choose to sit or to stand at any time. |
| "If you are seated … If you are standing …" | Cueing both options normalizes changing positions and makes all feel a part of the group. |
| "When you are ready …"<br>"If you like …"<br>(From David Emerson's *Overcoming Trauma Through Yoga*) | These phrases offer continuing choices that empower and ground in the present.<br>"Am I ready?" "Do I want to?" |
| "Give yourself a moment (or time) to …" | The word 'give' can empower someone to practice self-care. |
| "It's body physiology." | This simple phrase reinforces the idea that there is biology behind some actions and feelings. It can take 'guilt out of the equation.' (See p.6 for Dr. Ratey's quote.) |
| "Always move in a way that feels comfortable to you *today*."<br>"Even small stretches have benefits." | Offering at various time throughout a practice is a gentle reminder there are no expectations. |
| "The suggestion is to practice 'Feel the Breath' 3 times." | Putting a number boundary on a flow can help expand windows of tolerance. Someone also can gauge personal growth. |
| "The suggestion is to practice the 'Tip-to-Toe' stretch 3 times." | Naming a pose/breath/stretch provides predictability. "Oh, I know this." It also allows someone to easily think of it later. |
| "You can come out of this stretch (put your foot down) any time; you are never stuck." | Offering before a challenging pose can build the sense of safety needed to try new things. |
| "Different days, different stretches." | This phrase normalizes making a choice, supports curiosity, and improves a sense of time. |
| "We always do both sides." | Offer at beginning of a pose to prevent distraction of wondering if you will do both sides or which side someone should be on. |
| "Find a way to do this pose that makes you feel strong today." | Offer during a more challenging pose. |
| "The suggestion is …" | Use often to reinforce the idea that you are simply offering suggestions. |
| "Choose the pieces of the stretch that feel comfortable to you today." | Offer in a sequential stretch (seated cat/cow). |
| "*Today* you may want to put your hand on the chair to focus on the stretch. Or today you may want to take your hand off the chair and focus on building core." | Normalize using a chair. |
| "*Today* you can move with me or find your own stretches today." | Offer with any open-ended stretches and a reminder that each day can be different. |

**Table 11.2** Phrases to Build Body Awareness

| Trauma-informed Phrase | When/Why to Use |
|---|---|
| "Notice where you feel the stretch *today*." | A gentle reminder to notice is appropriate throughout the practice. |
| "Move until you feel yourself 'finding your balance'." | Offer to normalize movement (wobbling) to support someone physically experiencing 'finding their balance'. |
| "When you are ready, gently press one shoulder back … Then, press the other shoulder back." | Offer to the *entire* group if you notice someone slumping. |
| "You may like to move so that you feel a stretch across your shoulder blades today." | Offer as a guide in open-ended stretches. |
| "When you notice the muscles in your arms (or legs) … when you notice the muscles in your arms (or legs) … wiggle your fingers," OR press on your toes OR make gentle fists OR turn your palms up." | Suggest ONLY one of these cues in a strengthening pose. |
| "Move in any way that makes you smile." | Offer when a sense of play is needed (challenging balance poses). |
| "Find you own rhythm if you like: As YOU breathe in, press down on your hands (or toes …). As YOU breathe out … release …" | Offering in a pose that is *not* challenging (seated twist or lying down) supports focus on the rhythm of breath and movement. |
| "Find your own rhythm as you move from side to side" | Offer in any pose with movement. ('Tip-to-Toe' or wide-legged add-on) |
| "If you like, put one or both hands over your heart. When you feel your heart beating … when you feel your heart beathing, switch hands." | Offer the suggestion after moving. It can be disconcerting to not feel your resting heartbeat. |
| "'Take up Space' as you practice longer breaths in, fingers stretched wide. Maybe even your toes stretch wide." | Offer at the end of 'Final Stretch' or as an option to come out of eagle pose or tree pose. |
| "If you like, gently *move* the fingers on one hand or shake that hand … Then gently *move* the fingers on the other hand or shake that hand." | This cue ends all breathwork and can be added to a flow when you notice someone needs to ground. |

**Table 11.3** Phrases to Build Breath Awareness

| Trauma-informed Phrase | When/Why to Use |
|---|---|
| "When you are ready, gently press one shoulder back … Then, press the other shoulder back." | Offer before all breathwork. It signals breathwork is worthy of a setup. It may become a habit to take home. |
| "As YOU breathe in … As YOU breathe out …" or "On YOUR next breath in …" | Cueing every breath with emphasis on YOU supports someone practicing ways to manage their breath. |
| The suggestion is to practice 'The Wave Breath' 5 times. | A time boundary on breathwork allows someone to focus on the breathing, not on wondering how long it will last. |
| "Long, slow breaths out *can* lower heart rate, lower blood pressure, and lower muscle tension." | Offer in some breathwork cues to support someone making a choice about how to breathe. |
| "Longer breaths in *can* be energizing." | Offer before any breath when you observe someone seems tired or collapsed, or at the end of a practice to transition to rest of day. |
| "Find a place where it is easy to breathe." | Offer in a more challenging pose. |
| "When you notice you are breathing … when you notice you are breathing, wiggle your fingers." | Offer in a challenging pose when someone might be holding their breath. (tree pose, warriors, eagle) |
| "Always breathe in a comfortable way." | Use as a gentle reminder throughout the practice. |
| "Take your time with your words … Take your time with your breath … Don't rush your words … Don't rush your breath." | When familiar with a 5-part breathwork, cue it (2 or 3) times. "Now if you'd like, say it to yourself (2 or 3) times in your mind because you are always with you." You can keep talking to avoid dead air. |

## Two-to-Five Minute Breaks

These short breathing and movement breaks can change what Stephen Porges calls the physiological platform. Quite simply, these breaks can help turn it around. Based on body physiology, three formats in Table 11.4 are designed to energize, to calm, or to ground. They include: 1) two minutes: one breathing or simple stretching break; 2) three-to-four minutes: one breathing and one simple stretching break; and 3) four-to-five-minutes: one breathing break, one simple stretching break, and another breathing break. Again, download the scripts, MP3s, MP4s, and handouts to support your teaching.

**Table 11.4** Two-to-Five-Minute Breaks

| Breath fact To share | Breaks 1 A-C: 2 Minutes | Breaks 2 A-C: 3-4 Minutes | Breaks 3 A-C: 4-to-5 Minutes |
|---|---|---|---|
| **To Energize** Longer breaths in *can* be energizing. | **Break 1A. (2:27)** 3 Shoulder Rolls Back 'Feel the Breath' | **Break 2A. (3:26)** Tip-to-Toe' Stretch 'Finger Stretch Breath' | **Break 3A. (5:07)** 'Tip-to-Toe' Stretch The Chair Flow Balance 'The Wave Breath' |
| **To Calm** Long, slow breaths out *can* lower blood pressure. | **Break 1B. (2:56)** Seated Cat/Cow 'Finger Press Breath' | **Break 2B. (4:16)** Seated Twist with Cat/Cow Seated Circles | **Break 3B. (5:26)** Wide-legged Add-on 'Goal Post Breathing' 'It's a Wrap Breath' |
| **To Ground** Long, slow breaths out *can* lower heart rate. | **Break 1C. (2:18)** 'Shifting Breaths' | **Break 2C. (4:18)** 'Shifting Breaths' w/ Balance 'Open/Close Breath' ('Fist') | **Break 3C. and 3D.** 3C. Eagle Pose and 'Choose a Breathing Pattern' **(5:30)** 3D. Tree Pose and 'Choose a Breathing Pattern' **(5:00)** |

## Five Practice Sequences (30–90 Minutes)

These five practice sequences address specific trauma recovery considerations and are outlined in Table 11.5.

I. **'Feel the Flow' (30 minutes):** This sequence supports the somatic experience of flowing in and out of feeling states (effort and ease) by pairing simple breathwork with movement. The flows allow someone to experience and then to practice not being stuck (p. 194).

II. **Building Core (30 minutes):** This sequence supports the somatic experience of 'finding your balance' and building physical strength (p. 200).

III. **'Play it By Ear' (30 minutes):** This sequence focuses on the hearing modality to guide a somatic experience by creating opportunities simply to listen. Yet it includes the option of visual cues. It can be used as 'Self-care for Screen Fatigue' (p. 205).

IV. **Stretch and Strengthen with Balance (60–90 minutes):** This sequence builds self-regulation skills through simple stretching, gentle strengthening, and simple breathwork to empower and to challenge (p. 211).

V. **'All Together Now' (60 minutes):** This sequence supports refugee and immigrant (ESOL) groups building connection with themselves and their communities (p. 220).

**Table 11.5** 30-to-90-Minutes

I. 'Feel the Flow' (30 minutes)

A. STANDING

1. 'Shifting Breaths'
2. Wide-legged Add-on w/ Toe Stretches
3. 'Feel the Breath'
4. The Chair Pose Flow

B. SEATED

1. Comfortable Seat
2. Shoulder Stretches

    a.  The '1-2-3' Stretch
    b.  'Goal Post' Breathing w/ 'It's a Wrap'
    c.  'Shoulder Rock 'n Roll'

3. 'Finger Press Breath'

C. STANDING (by chair)

1. Hip Stretches

    a.  Pendulum/ Circle/ Toe Stretches
    b.  Eagle Pose Flow
    c.  'Take Up Space'
    d.  Wrap-Up

Side 1: Feel Heartbeat/Toe Stretches
Side 2: Toe Stretches/'Feel the Breath'

D. SEATED
1. Comfortable Seat
2. 'Stop Sign Breath'

E. 'Make a Plan'

II. Building Core (30 minutes)

A. STANDING

1. 'Tip-to-Toe' w/ Balance
2. Toe Stretches
3. 'Shifting Breaths' w/ Balance

B. STANDING (by chair)

1. Hip Stretches

    a.  Pendulum/Circle/Toe Stretches
    b.  Warrior Three
    c.  'Finger Press Breath'
    d.  Tree Pose w/ Toe Stretches

2. 'Feel the Breath'

-w/ choose breathing pattern

C. SEATED

1. Comfortable Seat
2. Shoulder Rolls
3. 'Find a New Stretch'
4. 'Fist Breathing' ('Open and Close Breath')

D. 'Make a Plan'

III. 'Play It by Ear' (30 minutes)

A. SEATED

1. Comfortable Seat
2. 'Feel the Breath'
3. Shoulder Stretches

    a.  The '1-2-3' Stretch
    b.  Shoulder Rolls
    c.  'Find a New Stretch'

B. STANDING

1. 'Tip-to-Toe'
2. Toe Stretches
3. 'Ring the Bell'
4. Wide-legged Add-on
5. 'Shifting Breath' with Balance

C. STANDING

1. 'Kitchen Stretch' (behind chair)

Set up

    a.  'Strong and Steady'
    b.  'Hip Rock 'n Roll
    c.  'Strong and Steady'
    d.  Shoulder Rolls Back

2. 'Tip-to-Toe' Stretch
3. 'Ring the Bell'

D. SEATED

1. Comfortable Seat
2. 'Feel the Breath' w/ choose breathing pattern
3. Classic Twist and Cat/Cow
4. Anytime/Anywhere' Breath

E. 'Make a Plan'

**IV: Stretch and Strengthen with Balance (60 minutes)**

**A. STANDING**

1. 'Tip-to-Toe' Stretch w/ Balance
2. Toe Stretches
3. 'Shifting Breaths' w/ Leg Balance
4. Wide-legged Add-on with Balance
5. 'Ring the Bell'
6. 'Feel the Breath'
7. Chair Flow Balance
8. The 'Finger Press Breath' (3x)
9. Warrior Two Flow
10. The 'Finger Press Breath' (3x)

**B. STANDING (by chair)**

1. Strengthening Flows (a/b)

    a. Warrior 3
    b. 'The Finger Press Breath'
    c. Tree Pose

**V. 'All Together Now' (Refugee/Immigrant/ESOL 60 minutes)**

**A. OPENING CONNECTIONS (10 minutes)**

**B. STANDING**

1. 'Silly Shake and Stretch'
2. 'Feel the Breath'
3. 'Tip-to-Toe' Stretch
4. 'Ring the Bell'
5. Wide-legged Add-on
6. Toe Stretches

**C. SEATED**

1. Comfortable Seat
2. 'Feel the Breath'
3. Neck and Shoulder Stretches

    a. Neck Massage
    b. Lift and Release Chin
    c. Shoulder Rolls
    d. 'The 1-2-3' Stretch

4. 'Open and Close' Breath

**D. STANDING**

1. Peaceful Warrior with Counting
2. 'Feel the Breath'

Side 1: Arms Open/#4 with Twist/'Take up Space'/Feel Heartbeat/Toe Stretch
Side 2: Arms Flowing/Shoulder Rolls/ #4 with Twist/ 'Take up Space'/ Toe Stretch

2. "Feel the Breath' choose breathing pattern
3. 'Tip-to-Toe' Stretch w/ Balance

**C. SEATED**

1. Comfortable Seat
2. 'Wave Breath'
3. Seated Shoulder Stretches

    a. The '1-2-3' Stretch
    b. Shoulder Rolls
    c. Find a New Stretch

4. Twist with Cat/Cow

**D. 'FINAL STRETCH' (15 minutes)**

1. 'Get Set Up'
2. 'Final Stretch'
3. 'Make a Plan'

3. Find a New Stretch

**E. STANDING (by chair)**

1. Tree Pose w/ Toe Stretch
2. 'Kitchen Stretch'

Setup

    a. 'Strong and Steady'
    b. 'Hip Rock 'n Roll'
    c. Shoulder Rolls Back

3. 'Ring the Bell'
4. 'Tip-to-Toe'

**F. SEATED**

1. Comfortable Seat
2. 'Wave Breath'
3. Favorites
4. Classic Twist with Cat/Cow

**G. 'Make a Plan**

## Three 30-Minute Practice Scripts

I. 'Feel the Flow' (30 minutes): This sequence supports the somatic experience of flowing in and out of feeling states (effort and ease) by linking simple breathwork and movement. The flow allows someone to experience and then to practice not being stuck (p. 194).

## A. Standing

Anything that we do standing, you can do seated or even lying down. You can always find ways to breathe and move with me.

1.  'Shifting Breaths' (more on p. 194) (photos p. 242 (a) and (b))

    1)  "When you are ready, gently press one shoulder back ... Then press the other shoulder back. The suggestion is to practice 3 'Shifting Breaths' with your palms forward.

    As YOU breathe in, shift forward. ... As YOU breathe out, release. (*Say 3 times slowly.*)

    2)  Now let's practice 3 'Shifting Breaths' with palms facing back. Keeping a gentle bend in your knees can protect your knee joints.

    As YOU breathe in, shift back ... As YOU breathe out, release. (*Say 3 times slowly.*)

    3)  If you like, gently *stretch* the fingers on one hand or shake that hand ... Then gently *stretch* the fingers on the other hand or shake that hand. Let your hands be as still as you would like them to be."

    **Variation:** "As YOU breathe in, palms forward, shift forward, today your *heels* may lift ... As YOU breathe out, release. Notice if you have a slight bend in your knees. On YOUR next breath in, palms back, shift back, *toes* lift ... As YOU breathe out, release." (*Say 3 times slowly.*)

2.  Wide-legged Add-ons with Toes Stretches (photos p. 234 (a)–(c))

    1)  "When you are ready, step your feet apart, hands on your hips.
    2)  If you like, roll from the inside edges to the outside edges of your feet ... Roll from the inside to the outside edges of your feet.
    3)  In a way that feels comfortable for you today, press one hip to one side ... Then press the other hip to the other side. Find your own rhythm as you move.

4) Perhaps gently lift and then arc one shoulder as you press your hip to one side ... Then gently lift and arc the other shoulder as you press to the other side.

5) Come back to standing tall, hands on your hips.

6) When you are ready, gently press one shoulder back ... Then press the other shoulder back.

7) If you like, lift one heel and press on the toes in a comfortable way. Then lift the other heel and press on the toes. The suggestion is to practice 2 more sets of toe stretches." (*Say 2 times slowly.*)

**Variation:** Perhaps today as you move from side to side, arc one arm overhead, fingers spread wide ... Then arc the other arm overhead, fingers spread wide.

3. **'Feel The Breath'** (more on p. 125)

1) "When you are ready, gently press one shoulder back ... Then press the other shoulder back.

2) (*Your choice of breath fact to share.*)

3) If you like, put one or both hands over your heart ... Put one or both hands over your heart.

4) The suggestion is to practice 5 breaths. Feel the breath in ... Feel the breath out. (*Say 2 times slowly.*) Always breathe in a comfortable way. Feel the breath in ... Feel the breath out. (*Say 3 times slowly.*)

5) If you like, gently *stretch* the fingers on one hand or shake that hand ... Then gently *stretch* the fingers on the other hand or shake that hand. Let your hands be as still as you would like them to be."

4. **The Chair Pose Flow** (photos p. 236 (a)–(e))

**Warm-up:** "The suggestion is to practice the chair flow warm-up 3 times.

As YOU breathe in, look up, stretch up, *fingertips* press overhead ... As YOU breathe out, arms release, *fingertips* tap your sides."
(*Say three times slowly.*)

**Variation:** 1st breath: *fingertips* press; 2nd breath: *palms* press; 3rd breath: Your choice: *fingertips* or *palms* press.

**The Chair Pose Flow**

1) "Today you may want to bend your knees as we practice the chair flow 3 times.

2) As YOU breathe in, look up, stretch up, *fingertips* press overhead …
As YOU breathe out, knees bend in a comfortable way, arms release,
fingers spread wide." (*Say 3 times slowly.*)

**Variation:** 3rd breath: "The suggestion is to pause halfway down and find
a place to hold the stretch. Wherever you pause, hold the stretch … but
not your breath. Let's practice two more breaths here. Feel the breath in
… Feel the breath out." (*Say 2 times slowly.*)

## B. Seated

1. **Comfortable Seat**

   1) "Give yourself a few moments to find a comfortable way to sit today,
      either on a chair or the floor, perhaps on a folded blanket or cushion.
   2) When you are ready, gently press one shoulder back … Then press
      the other shoulder back.
   3) If you like, move from side to side as you find a comfortable seat. You
      may want to move in a circle. Give yourself time as you move. If you
      like, circle the other way.
   4) Make any adjustments to make your seat more comfortable.
   5) If you like, tap your *hands or feet* 4 times."

2. **Shoulder Stretches (a./b./c.)**

   a. **The '1-2-3' Shoulder Stretch** (photo on p. 239 (a)–(c))

      1) "When you are ready, gently bend your elbows in a comfortable
         way as we practice the '1-2-3' shoulder stretch.
      2) As you breathe in, press both shoulders back. That's 1.

      As you breathe out, press both shoulders forward. That's 2. And
      release. That's 3.

      3) The suggestion is to practice two more sets of the '1-2-3' shoulder
         stretch. (*Say slowly 2 more times.*)
      4) If you like, tap your *feet* 4 times."

   b. **'Goal Post Breathing' with 'It's a Wrap'** (photo on p. 241 (a)–(c))

      1) **'Goal Post Breathing'**

         1) "When you are ready, gently press one shoulder back …
            Then press the other shoulder back. (*No breath fact.*)

2)  The suggestion is to practice 'Goal Post Breathing' 5 times. With each breath in, you can move your hands farther apart in any way that is comfortable to you today.

As YOU breathe in, hands apart … As YOU breathe out, fingertips press. As YOU breathe in, hands a little farther apart … As YOU breathe out, fingertips press.

Always breathe and move in a comfortable way.

On YOUR next breath in, hands a little farther apart … As YOU breathe out, fingertips press. As YOU breathe in, hands a little farther apart … As YOU breathe out, fingertips press." (*Repeat last cue slowly.*)

### 2) 'It's a Wrap'

1)  "Now if you like, create a comfortable arm wrap. (*No breath fact.*)
2)  The suggestion is to practice 3 breaths in 'It's a Wrap'. As YOU breathe in, fingers gently press … As YOU breathe out, release the press. (*Say 3 times slowly.*)
3)  If you like, create a wrap with the other arm on top. **(Repeat.)**
4)  When you are ready, gently *move* the fingers on one hand or shake that hand … Then gently *move* the fingers on the other hand or shake that hand."

### c.  'Shoulder Rock 'n Roll' (photo on p. 239 (d))

1)  "When you are ready, gently bend your elbows and stretch your fingers in a comfortable way.
2)  If you like, move one arm across the front and the other arm across the back as we practice 'Shoulder Rock 'n Roll'. Now move the other arm across the front, and the other across the back. That's 1 set. The suggestion is to find your own rhythm as we practice 2 more sets." (*Say 3 times slowly.*)

## 3.  The 'Finger Press Breath' (see p. 126)

1)  "When you are ready, gently press one shoulder back … Then press the other shoulder back.
2)  (*Your choice of breath fact to share.*)
3)  If you like, put one or both hands over your heart … Put one or both hands over your heart.
4)  The suggestion is to practice the 'Finger Press Breath' three times. As YOU breathe in, fingers press … As YOU breathe out, release the press. (*Say 3 times slowly.*)

5) If you like, gently *move* the fingers on one hand or shake that hand … Then *move* the fingers on the other hand or shake that hand. Let your hands be as still as you would like them to be."

## C. Standing (by chair)

Anything that we do standing, you can do seated or even lying down. You can always find ways to stretch and breathe with me.

1. **Hip Stretches: (Side 1: a./b./c./d. and Side 2: a./b./c./d.)**

   a. **Pendulum and Circle with Toe Stretch (photos p. 234 (a) and (b))**

      1) "We always do both sides. When you are ready, stand by your chair. The suggestion is to slowly move your leg from side to side. A slight bend in your standing leg can protect your knee joint.
      2) As you move to 'find your balance', you are building core muscles. With your hand on the chair, you are focusing on the stretch.
      3) When you are ready, move your leg in a circle, a spiral, or any comfortable way. Then perhaps move it even more slowly.
      4) Notice if you smile as you take your hand off the chair to 'find your balance'. When you are ready, circle your leg in the other direction. Give yourself time with the stretch.
      5) When you are ready, stand tall with your hands on your hips.
      6) If you like, lift one heel and press on the toes. Then lift the other heel and press on the toes. The suggestion is to practice two more sets of toe stretches." (*Say 2 more times slowly.*)

   **Variation:** You may want to move your leg in a *new* way today.

   b. **Eagle Pose (photos p. 229)**

      1) "When you are ready, move one leg forward and around your standing leg as we practice eagle pose. Find a way to stand that makes you feel strong today. Your toes can be on the floor, pressing against your standing leg, or wrapping around that leg. Different days, different stretches.
      2) The top part of eagle can be done with one or both hands over your heart. Or today you could put one elbow over the other. Notice if it is comfortable to lift your elbows. Give yourself a few moments to find your eagle pose for today.
      3) You can always put your foot down; you are never stuck. Notice if bending your knees changes the stretch.

4)   To come out of eagle, either stand tall with your hands over your heart or 'Take Up Space'."

c.   **'Take Up Space' (Half-Moon)** (photos p. 230 (a) and (b))

"With your hand on or off the chair, practice longer breaths in if that is comfortable, spread your fingers wide … extend your leg out to the side … as you breathe and stretch and strengthen. The suggestion is to practice 2 more longer breaths in. On YOUR next breath in, stretch out and 'take up space'. As YOU breathe out, *wiggle* your fingers or toes. (*Say 2 times slowly.*) When you are ready and as *slowly* as you would like, release to standing tall."

d.   **Hip Stretch Wrap-up**

**Side 1: (1) Feel the Heartbeat.** "When you are ready, put one or both hands over your heart. When you feel your heart beating … when you feel your heart beating, switch hands."

**(2) Toe Stretches.** "If you like, put your hands on your hips. Lift one heel and press on the toes in a comfortable way. Then lift the other heel and press on the toes. The suggestion is to practice 2 more sets of toe stretches." (*Say 2 times slowly.*) **(Standing on the other side of the chair, repeat a./b./c./d. on side 2.)**

**Side 2: (1) Toe Stretches (2) 'Feel the Breath'** (See p. 195.)

## D. Seated

1.   **Comfortable Seat** (see above)

2.   **'Stop Sign Breath'** (more on pp. 137/199–200) (photos on p. 241 (d) and (e))

1)   "When you are ready, gently press one shoulder back … Then press the other shoulder back.
2)   (*No breath fact.*) The suggestion is to practice the 'Stop Sign Breath' 5 times.

As YOU breathe in, palms press forward, (ONLY *you softly say* 'stop') … As YOU breathe out, fingers down. (*Say 2 times slowly.*) Always move and breathe in a comfortable way.

On YOUR next breath in, palms press forward, (*stop*) … As YOU breathe out, fingers down.

As YOU breathe in, palms forward, (*stop*) … As YOU breathe out, fingers down. (*Repeat last cue slowly.*)

3) If you like, gently *wiggle* the finger on one hand or shake that hand, then gently *wiggle* the fingers on the other hand or shake that hand."

## E. 'Make a Plan'

1) "Give yourself a few moments to make a 2-minute plan to use later when you want to change how you are feeling. You can interrupt your stress cycle by managing how you breathe and move.
2) The suggestion is to choose one breath we did today: we did the 'Feel the Breath', 'Shifting Breaths', and 'Stop Sign Breath'. Longer breaths out *can* lower blood pressure. So now you have a one-minute breath to practice.
3) If you like, add one stretch, perhaps the wide-legged add-on or the '1-2-3' shoulder stretch. You now have a two-minute plan to do at home or at work when you want to change how you are feeling."

**To Extend: After D, repeat Seated Shoulder Stretches.**

**II. Building Core (30 minutes): This sequence supports the somatic experience of 'finding your balance' and building physical strength.**

## A. Standing

Anything that we do standing, you can do seated or even lying down. You can always find ways to stretch and breathe with me.

1. **'Tip-to-Toe' Stretch with Balance** (photos p. 231)

    1) "When you are ready, stretch one arm to the side or overhead as we do the 'Tip-to-Toe' stretch. Then stretch the other arm to the side or overhead.
    2) Find your own rhythm as you stretch one arm, fingers spread wide … Then stretch the other arm, fingers spread wide.
    3) If you like, lift one leg to the side in a comfortable way. As you 'find your balance', you are building core. Let's practice 2 more breaths. Feel the breath in … Feel the breath out. (*Say 2 times slowly.*)
    4) When you are ready, come back to standing tall, hands on your hips. **(Repeat on the other side.)** Notice if finding your balance *feels* different on the second side."

2. **Toe Stretches**

    1) "When you are ready, gently press one shoulder back … Then press the other shoulder back.

2) If you like, lift one heel and press on the toes in a comfortable way. Then lift the other heel and press on the toes. The suggestion is to practice two more sets of toe stretches. (*Say two more times slowly.*)

**Variation:** Lift a heel ... press on the toes ... roll over the toes ... and gently press. If you like, lift the other heel ... press on the toes ... roll over the toes ... and gently press. That's one set. Notice if you want to press more firmly or more gently as we practice two more sets of toe stretches." (*Say 2 more times slowly.*)

3. **'Shifting Breaths' with Balance** (photos p. 242 (a) and (b))

1) "When you are ready, gently press one shoulder back ... Then press the other shoulder back. The suggestion is to practice 3 'Shifting Breaths' with your palms forward.

As YOU breathe in, shift forward, today your *heels* may lift. ... As YOU breathe out, release. (*Say 3 times slowly.*)

2) Now let's practice 3 'Shifting Breaths' with palms facing back. Keeping a gentle bend in your knees can protect your knee joints. As YOU breathe in, shift back, today your *toes* may lift ... As YOU breathe out, release. (*Say 3 times slowly.*)

3) When you are ready, come back to standing tall. If you like, gently *stretch* the fingers on one hand or shake that hand ... Then gently *stretch* the fingers on the other hand or shake that hand."

## B. Standing (by chair)

Anything that we do standing, you can do seated as well.

1. **Hip Stretches: (Side 1: a./b./c./d./e. and Side 2: a./b./c./d./e.)** (photos p. 234 (a) and (b))

a. **Pendulum and Circle and Toe Stretches**

1) "We always do both sides. When you are ready, stand by your chair. The suggestion is to slowly move your leg from side to side. A slight bend in your standing leg can protect that knee joint.

2) As you move to 'find your balance', you are building core muscles. With your hand on the chair, you may be focusing on the stretch.

3) When you are ready, move your leg in a circle, a spiral, or any comfortable way. Now perhaps move it even more slowly.

4) Notice if you smile as you take your hand off the chair to 'find your balance'. When you are ready, circle your leg in the other direction. Give yourself time with the stretch.

5) When you are ready, stand tall with your hands on your hips.

6) If you like, lift one heel and press on the toes in a comfortable way. Then lift the other heel and press on the toes. The suggestion is to practice 2 more sets of toe stretches." (*Say 2 more times slowly.*)

**Variation:** You may want to move your leg in a *new* way today.

b. **Warrior Three** (photos p. 235)

1) "When you are ready, put one hand on the chair. Extend your leg back to create the stretch you want today. Perhaps today extend one or both arms forward.

2) You can put your foot down anytime; you are never stuck. If you like, hold the stretch … but not your breath. Let's practice 2 more breaths here. Feel the breath in … Feel the breath out. (*Say 2 times slowly.*)

3) When you notice your leg muscles working … when you notice your leg muscles working, **(Side 1):** *wiggle* your fingers. **(Side 2):** *press* on your toes.

4) When you are ready, come back to standing tall."

c. **The 'Finger Press Breath'**

1) "When you are ready, gently press one shoulder back … Then press the other shoulder back.

2) (*Your choice of breath fact to share.*)

3) If you like, put one or both hands over your heart … Put one or both hands over your heart.

4) The suggestion is to practice the 'Finger Press Breath' 3 times. As YOU breathe in, fingers press … As YOU breathe out, release the press. (*Say 3 times slowly.*)

5) If you like, gently *move* the fingers on one hand or shake that hand … Then *move* the fingers on the other hand or shake that hand. Let your hands be as still as you would like them to be."

d. **Tree Pose** (photos p. 228 (a)–(f))

**Setup:** 1) "When you are ready, turn your knee open and press your foot against your standing leg so that you feel *strong* today. But pressing your foot on your knee can put pressure on your knee joint.

2) Today you may want your hand on the chair. When you take it off the chair, notice how you are 'finding your balance'. You can put your foot down any time; you are never stuck.

**Side 1:** The suggestion is to practice 3 breaths. As YOU breathe in, one or both arms open wide, fingers stretch. As YOU breathe out, hands over your heart. (*Say 3 times slowly.*)

**Side 2:** If you like, stretch one or both arms to the side or overhead. Move your arms in any way that makes you smile. You can move with me or find your own ways to *play* with balance. Today you may move your arms in a new way, simply noticing how they are moving."

**Variation:** "If you haven't tried to 'find your balance' today, perhaps move in a way to 'find your balance' now. You can put your foot down anytime and then try it again."

e. **Toe Stretches**

1) "The suggestion is to come back to standing tall, hands on your hips.
2) When you are ready, gently press one shoulder back ... Then press the other shoulder back.
3) If you like, lift one heel and press on the toes in a way that feels comfortable today. Then lift the other heel and press on the toes. The suggestion is to practice 2 more sets of toe stretches." (*Say 2 times slowly.*) **(Repeat Side 2: a./b./c./d./e.)**

2. **'Feel the Breath' – Choose Your Breathing Pattern**

1) "When you are ready, gently press one shoulder back ... Then press the other shoulder back.
2) Long, slow breaths out *can* lower blood pressure and lower heart rate. Longer breaths in *can* be energizing.
3) If you like, put one or both hands over your heart ... Put one or both hands over your heart. The suggestion is to practice 5 breaths with the breathing pattern you choose.
4) Feel the breath in ... Feel the breath out. (*Say 2 times slowly.*) Always breathe in a comfortable way. Feel the breath in ... Feel the breath out. (*Say 3 times slowly.*)
5) If you like, gently *stretch* the fingers on one hand or shake that hand ... Then gently *stretch* the fingers on the other hand or shake that hand."

## C. Seated

1. **Comfortable Seat**

    1) "Give yourself a few moments to find a comfortable way to sit today, either on a chair or the floor, perhaps on a folded blanket or cushion.
    2) If you like, move from side to side as you find a comfortable seat. You may want to move in a circle. Give yourself time as you move. If you like, circle the other way.
    3) Make any adjustments to make your seat more comfortable.
    4) When you are ready, gently press one shoulder back ... Then press the other shoulder back.
    5) If you like, tap your *fingertips* 4 times."

2. **Shoulder Rolls** (photos p. 238)

    1) "The suggestion is to practice 3 shoulder rolls forward and 3 back.
    2) As YOU breathe in, shoulders lift ... As YOU breathe out, shoulders roll forward and down. (*Say 3 times slowly.*)
    3) As YOU breathe in, shoulders lift ... As YOU breathe out, shoulders roll back and down." (*Say 3 times slowly.*)

3. **'Find a New Stretch'**

    1) "Give yourself a few moments to find a *new* way to stretch. You can move with me or perhaps find your own *new* way to move today. (*Slowly cue all your stretches.*)
    2) If you like, tap your *hands* on your legs 4 times. Then move your hands 4 times in a new way – perhaps strumming or patting."

4. **'Fist Breathing' ('Open and Close Breath')** (more on p. 127)

    1) "When you are ready, gently press one shoulder back ... Then press the other shoulder back.
    2) The suggestion is to try one or more of these four ways to move your fingers with me now. (*Say slowly as you do each one as a group.*) The first is moving your fingers a small amount. Another way is pressing four fingers on your thumbs. Or today you might gently press your fingers on your palms. The last suggestion is to make tight fists, maybe so tight you feel your forearms and face tighten.
    3) (*Your choice of breath fact to share.*)
    4) If you like, choose one way to move your fingers as we practice 'Fist Breathing' ('Open and Close Breathing') 5 times.

As YOU breathe in, fingers move … As YOU breathe out, release. (*Say 2 times slowly.*)

Always breathe and move in a comfortable way.

On YOUR next breath in, fingers move … As YOU breathe out, release.

As YOU breathe in, fingers move … As YOU breathe out, release. (*Repeat last cue slowly.*)

5) If you like, gently *wiggle* the fingers on one hand or shake that hand … Then gently *wiggle* the fingers on the other hand or shake that hand."

**Variation:** "Today you may like to try moving your fingers in a *new* way, one you haven't done before."

## D. 'Make a Plan'

1) "Give yourself a few moments to make a 2-minute plan to use later when you want to change how you are feeling. You can interrupt your stress cycle by managing how you breathe.
2) The suggestion is to choose one breath we did today: we did 'Shifting Breaths', 'Feel the Breath', and 'Fist Breathing' ('Open and Close Breath'). Long, slow breaths out *can* lower blood pressure.
3) If you like, add one stretch – perhaps shoulder rolls or tree pose.
4) You now have a two-minute plan to do at home or at work when you want to change how you are feeling."

**To Extend: After D, repeat A. Standing a./b./c.**

**III. 'Play It by Ear' (30 minutes): This sequence focuses on the hearing modality to guide the somatic experience by creating opportunities simply to listen. Yet it includes the option of visual cues. It can be used as 'Self-care for Screen/Zoom Fatigue'.**

Anything that we do standing, you can do seated or even lying down. You can always find ways to breathe and move with me.

## A. Seated

1. **Comfortable Seat**

1) "Give yourself a few moments to find a comfortable way to sit today, either on the floor or a chair. If you sit on the floor, perhaps sit on a folded blanket or cushion.

2) If you like, move from side to side as you find a comfortable seat. You may want to move in a circle. Give yourself time as you move. If you like, circle the other way.

3) Make any adjustments to make your seat more comfortable.

4) When you are ready, gently press one shoulder back … Then press the other shoulder back.5) If you like, tap your *fingertips* 4 times."

2. **'Feel the Breath'** (more on p. 125)

1) "When you are ready, gently press one shoulder back again … Then press the other shoulder back.

2) (*Your choice of breath fact to share.*)

3) If you like, put one or both hands over your heart … Put one or both hands over your heart.

The suggestion is to practice 5 breaths.

4) Feel the breath in … Feel the breath out. (*Say 2 times slowly.*) Always breathe in a comfortable way. Feel the breath in … Feel the breath out. (*Say 3 times slowly.*)

5) If you like, gently *stretch* the fingers on one hand or shake that hand … Then gently *stretch* the fingers on the other hand or shake that hand. Let your hands be as still as you would like them to be."

3. **Seated Shoulder Stretches (a./b./c.)** (photos p. 239 (a)–(c))

a. **The '1-2-3' Shoulder Stretch**

1) "When you are ready, gently bend your elbows in a comfortable way as we practice the '1-2-3' shoulder stretch.

2) As you breathe in, press both shoulders back. That's 1.

As you breathe out, press both shoulders forward. That's 2. And release. That's 3.

3) The suggestion is to practice two more sets of the '1-2-3' shoulder stretch. (*Say slowly 3 more times.*)

4) If you like, tap your *hands or feet* 4 times."

b. **Shoulder Rolls**

1) "The suggestion is to practice 3 shoulder rolls forward and 3 back.

2) As YOU breathe in, shoulders lift … As YOU breathe out, shoulders roll forward and down. (*Say 3 times slowly.*)

3) As YOU breathe in, shoulders lift ... As YOU breathe out, shoulders roll back and down." (*Say 3 times slowly.*)

c. **'Find a New Stretch'**

1) "Give yourself a few moments to find a *new* stretch. You can move with me or perhaps find your own way to move today. (*Cue your stretches.*)

2) If you like, tap your *fingertips* on your legs 4 times. Then move your *fingertips* 4 times in a *new* way, perhaps strumming or patting."

## B. Standing

1. **'Tip-to-Toe' Stretch** (photos p. 231 (a)–(e))

1) "Anything that we do standing, you can do seated as well. When you are ready, stretch one arm to the side or overhead as we do the 'Tip-to-Toe' stretch. Then stretch the other arm to the side or overhead.

2) Find your own rhythm as you stretch one arm, fingers spread wide ... Then stretch the other arm, fingers spread wide.

3) If you like, grasp one wrist as you gently stretch forward overhead. When you are ready, grasp the other wrist as you gently stretch the other arm.

4) When you are ready, come back to standing tall, hands on your hips."

2. **Toe Stretches**

1) "When you are ready, gently press one shoulder back ... Then press the other shoulder back.

2) If you like, lift one heel and press on the toes in a comfortable way. Then lift the other heel and press on the toes. The suggestion is to practice 2 more sets of toe stretches." (*Say 2 more times slowly.*)

**Variation:** "Lift a heel ... press on the toes ... roll over the toes ... and gently press. If you like, lift the other heel ... press on the toes ... roll over the toes ... and gently press. That's one set. Now press more firmly or more gently as we practice 2 more sets of toe stretches." (*Say 2 more times slowly.*)

3. **'Ring the Bell'** (photos p. 232 (a)–(c))

1) "When you are ready, step your feet apart in a comfortable way.

2) The suggestion as we practice the 'Ring the Bell' is to move one arm across the front and one across your back ... tapping your lowback ...

your midback … and your upper back as you move up and down your back.

3) If you like, hold your hands in a *new* way: now either 'ring the bell' with an open palm or a closed hand. Give yourself time with the stretch as you gently create length in your spine."

4. **Wide-legged Add-ons** (photos p. 234 (a)–(c))

1) "When you are ready, with your feet still apart, put your hands on your hips.
2) If you like, roll from the inside edges to the outside edges of your feet … Roll from the inside to the outside edges of your feet.
3) In whatever way feels comfortable to you today, press one hip to one side … Then press the other hip to the other side. Find your own rhythm as you move.
4) Perhaps gently lift and then arc one shoulder as you press your hip to one side … Then gently lift and arc the other shoulder as you press to the other side.
5) When you are ready, come back to standing tall."

**Variation:** Perhaps today as you move from side to side, arc one arm overhead, fingers spread wide … Then arc the other arm overhead, fingers spread wide.

5. **'Shifting Breaths' with Balance** (see p. 242 (a) and (b))

1) "When you are ready, gently press one shoulder back … Then press the other shoulder back.

2) The suggestion is to practice 3 'Shifting Breaths' with your palms facing forward.

As YOU breathe in, shift forward, today one or both *heels* may lift … As YOU breathe out, release. (*Say 3 times slowly.*)

3) Now let's practice 3 'Shifting Breaths' with palms facing back. Keeping a gentle bend in your knees can protect your knee joints. As YOU breathe in, shift back … today your toes may lift … As YOU breathe out, release. (*Say 3 times slowly.*)
4) If you like, gently *stretch* the fingers on one hand or shake that hand … Then gently *stretch* the fingers on the other hand or shake that hand. Let your hands be as still as you would like them to be."

## C. Standing

1. **'Kitchen Stretch' (a./b./a./c.)** (behind chair) (photos p. 237)

   **Setup:** 1) "Let's practice 3 ways to protect your back anytime you bend forward:
   gently press shoulders back, hips back, and slightly bend knees.
   2) When you are ready, rest your hands or forearms on the back of the chair.
   Notice that your shoulders are back, hips are back, and knees are bent."

   a. **'Strong and Steady'**

   "The suggestion is to practice 'Strong and Steady' with 4 breaths. As YOU breathe in, feel the press on the chair … As YOU breathe out, hips press back in a comfortable way." (*Say 4 times slowly.*)

   b. **'Hip Rock 'n Roll'**

   1) "If you like, stand and put your hands on your hips. Give yourself a moment to practice lifting your tailbone and tucking your tailbone. Find your own rhythm as you lift and tuck in 'Hip Rock 'n Roll'. Now set up for 'Kitchen Stretch' again. (*Repeat Setup.*) On YOUR next breath in, tailbone lifts … As YOU breathe out, tailbone tucks as we practice 'Hip Rock 'n Roll'.

   2) You can adjust your feet anytime; you are never stuck. If you like, practice two more sets, finding your own rhythm as you breathe and move in a comfortable way." (*Say 2 times slowly.*)

   **(Repeat a. 'Strong and Steady'.)**

   c. **Shoulder Rolls Back**

   "When you are ready, come to standing tall. Let's practice 3 shoulder rolls back. As YOU breathe in, shoulders lift … As YOU breathe out, shoulders roll back and down. (*Say 3 times slowly.*) Perhaps next time you are in the kitchen or at work, give yourself one minute to practice 'Kitchen Stretch' for your back."

2. **'Tip-to-Toe' Stretch** (see p. 207)

3. **'Ring the Bell'** (see pp. 207–208)

## D. Seated

1.  **Comfortable Seat** (see above)

2.  **'Feel the Breath' – Choose Your Breathing Pattern**

    1)  "When you are ready, gently press one shoulder back … Then press the other shoulder back.
    2)  Long, slow breaths out *can* lower blood pressure and lower heart rate. Longer breaths in can be energizing.
    3)  If you like, put one or both hands over your heart … Put one or both hands over your heart. The suggestion is to practice 5 breaths with the breathing pattern you choose.
    4)  Feel the breath in … Feel the breath out. (*Say 2 times slowly.*) Always breathe in a comfortable way. Feel the breath in … Feel the breath out. (*Say 3 times slowly.*)
    5)  If you like, gently *stretch* the fingers on one hand or shake that hand … Then gently *stretch* the fingers on the other hand or shake that hand."

3.  **Classic Twist with Cat/Cow** (photos p. 230 (c)–(e))

    1)  "When you are ready, tap your *fingertips* on your legs four times.
    2)  We always do both sides. On YOUR next breath in, press down on your hands … As YOU breathe out, bring your hands around to one side to create a gentle twist.
    3)  The suggestion is to practice 3 breaths as you find your own rhythm: As YOU breathe in, hands press … As YOU breathe out, release the press. (*Say 3 times slowly*).
    4)  When you are ready, come back to facing front, hands on your legs. If you like, tap your *hands* 4 times.
    5)  Let's practice seated cat/cow 2 times before we twist to the other side. Always move and breathe in a comfortable way. As YOU breathe in, chin lifts … shoulders back … rock forward. As YOU breathe out, chin tucks … shoulders forward … rock back in a comfortable way. (*Say 2 times slowly.*)
    6)  When you are ready, come back to sitting tall."
        **(Repeat on other side.)**

4.  **The 'Anytime/Anywhere Breath'** (more on p. 130) (photo on p. 242 (f))

    1)  "You can do the 'Anytime, Anywhere Breath' seated or standing, eyes open eyes closed, in a group, even when you are talking with someone.

2) When you are ready, gently press one shoulder back ... Then press the other shoulder back. If you like, place one hand on your leg.

3) The suggestion is to practice long, slow breaths out if that is comfortable to you today.

4) Let's practice 5 breaths. As YOU breathe in, fingers press ... As YOU breathe out, release. (*Say 2 times slowly.*) Always breathe in a comfortable way. On YOUR next breath in, fingers press ... As YOU breathe out, release. As YOU breathe in, fingers press ... As YOU breathe out, release. (*Repeat last cue slowly.*)

5) When you are ready, gently *move* the fingers on one hand or shake that hand ... Then gently *move* the fingers on the other hand or shake that hand."

## E. 'Make a Plan'

1) "Give yourself a few moments to make a 2-minute plan to use later when you want to change how you are feeling. You can interrupt your stress cycle by managing how you breathe and move.

2) The suggestion is to choose one breath we did today: we did 'Feel the Breath', 'Shifting Breaths', and the 'Anytime/Anywhere Breath'. A long breath out *can* lower blood pressure.

3) If you like, add one stretch – perhaps the 'Kitchen Stretch' or the 'Tip-to-Toe' stretch.

You now have a two-minute plan to do at home or at work when you want to change how you are feeling."

**To Extend: After D, repeat** Wide-legged Add-on/Toe Stretches/ 'Shifting Breaths'.

## Two 60–90-Minute Practice Scripts

IV. Stretching and Strengthening with Balance (60–90 minutes): This sequence builds self-regulation skills through simple stretching, gentle strengthening, and simple breathwork to empower and to challenge.

## A. Standing

Anything that we do standing, you can do seated or even lying down. You can always find ways to breathe and move with me.

1.  **'Tip-to-Toe' Stretch with Leg Balance** (photos p. 231)

    1)  "When you are ready, stretch one arm out to the side or overhead as we do the 'Tip-to-Toe' stretch. Then stretch the other arm to the side or overhead.
    2)  Find your own rhythm as you stretch one arm, fingers spread wide … Then stretch the other arm, fingers spread wide.
    3)  If you like, lift one leg to the side. As you 'find your balance', you are building core. Let's practice two more breaths. Feel the breath in … Feel the breath out. (*Say 2 times slowly.*)
    4)  When you are ready, come back to standing tall, hands on your hips. **(Repeat on other side.)**
    5)  Notice if 'finding your balance' *felt* different on the second side."

2.  **Toe Stretches**

    1)  "When you are ready, gently press one shoulder back … Then press the other shoulder back.
    2)  If you like, lift one heel and press on the toes in a comfortable way. Then lift the other heel and press on the toes. The suggestion is to practice 2 more sets of toe stretches. (*Say 2 times slowly.*)

    **Variation:** Lift a heel … press on the toes … roll over the toes … and gently press. If you like, lift the other heel … press on the toes … roll over the toes … and gently press. That's one set. Press more firmly or more gently as we practice 2 more sets." (*Say 3 times slowly.*)

3.  **'Shifting Breaths' with Leg Balance** (photos p. 242 (a)–(b))

    1)  "When you are ready, gently press one shoulder back … Then press the other shoulder back. The suggestion is to practice three 'Shifting Breaths' with a leg balance.
    2)  If you like, step one foot forward and across, any distance, palms forward. You can always adjust your feet; you are never stuck.
    3)  As YOU breathe in, shift forward. As YOU breathe out, release. (*Say 3 times slowly.*)
    4)  When you are ready, come back to standing tall.
    5)  If you like, step the other foot forward and across, any distance. **(Repeat #3.)**
    6)  When you are ready, come back to standing tall. If you like, gently *stretch* the fingers on one hand or shake that hand … Then gently *stretch* the fingers on the other hand or shake that hand."

4.  **Wide-legged Add-on with Balance** (photos p. 234 (a)–(c))

    1)  "When you are ready, step your feet apart, hands on your hips.
    2)  If you like, roll from the inside edges to the outside edges of your feet … roll from the inside to the outside edges of your feet in a comfortable way.
    3)  In a way that feels comfortable to you today, press one hip to one side … Then press the other hip to the other side. Find your own rhythm as you move from side to side.
    4)  Perhaps gently lift and then arc one shoulder as you press your hip to one side … Then gently lift and arc the other shoulder as you press to the other side.
    5)  Perhaps today, you can play with 'finding your balance' by lifting one foot to the side. Notice if 'finding your balance' *feels* the same on both sides.
    6)  When you are ready, come back to standing tall."

5.  **'Ring the Bell'** (photos p. 232 (a)–(c))

    1)  "When you are ready, step your feet apart again in a comfortable way.
    2)  The suggestion as we practice the 'Ring the Bell' is to move one arm across the front and one across your back … tapping your low back … your mid-back … and your upper back as you move up and down your back.
    3)  If you like, hold your hands in a *new* way: now either 'ring the bell' with an open palm or a closed hand. Take your time with the stretch as you gently create length in your spine."

6.  **'Feel the Breath'**

    1)  "When you are ready, gently press one shoulder back … Then press the other shoulder back.
    2)  (*Your choice of breath fact to share.*)
    3)  If you like, put one or both hands over your heart … Put one or both hands over your heart.
    4)  The suggestion is to practice 5 breaths.

    Feel the breath in … Feel the breath out. (*Say 2 times slowly.*) Always breathe in a comfortable way. Feel the breath in … Feel the breath out. (*Say 3 times slowly.*)

    5)  If you like, gently *move* the fingers on one hand or shake that hand … Then gently *move* the fingers on the other hand or shake that hand. Let your hands be as still as you would like them to be."

7. **The Chair Flow Balance** (photos p. 236)

**Warm-up:**

1) "The suggestion is to practice the chair flow warm-up three times.

As YOU breathe in, look up, stretch up, *fingertips* press overhead … As YOU breathe out, arms release, *fingertips* tap your sides.

2) Today, you may like to add lifting one or both heels as we finish the chair flow warm-up." (*Say 2 more times slowly.*)

**The Chair Flow Balance:**

1) "The suggestion is to add bending the knees as we do the chair flow balance 3 times.
2) As YOU breathe in, look up, stretch up, *fingertips* press overhead … As YOU breathe out, knees bend in a comfortable way, arms release, fingers spread wide.
3) On YOUR next breath in, lift one or both heels as you look up, stretch up, *fingertips* press overhead … As YOU breathe out, knees bend in a comfortable way, arms release, fingers spread wide. Find your own rhythm as you breathe and move.
4) On YOUR next breath in, lift the other heel or both heels, look up, stretch up, *fingertips* press overhead … As YOU *keep breathing* in a comfortable way, the suggestion is to pause halfway down and find a place to hold the stretch. If today is a challenge day for you, perhaps keep your *heels* lifted as you squat and wrap your arms around your shins. Wherever you pause, hold the stretch … but not your breath. Let's practice 2 more breaths here. Feel the breath in … Feel the breath out. (*Say 2 times slowly.*)
5) When you are ready, come back to standing tall."

8. **The 'Finger Press Breath'**

1) "When you are ready, gently press one shoulder back … Then press the other shoulder back.
2) (*Your choice of breath fact to share.*)
3) If you like, put one or both hands over your heart … Put one or both hands over your heart.
4) The suggestion is to practice the 'Finger Press Breath' 3 times. As YOU breathe in, fingers press … As YOU breathe out, release the press. (*Say 3 times slowly.*)

5) If you like, gently *move* the fingers on one hand or shake that hand … Then gently *move* the fingers on the other hand or shake that hand. Let your hands be as still as you would like them to be."

9. **Warrior Two Flow (Side 1: a./b./c./d. and Side 2: a./b./c./d.)** (photos p. 233)

   a.  **Warrior Two**

   **Setup:**  1) "We always do both sides. When you are ready, step one foot back. Notice if the back edge of your foot *feels* parallel to the back edge of the mat. Then perhaps look back and adjust.
2) Tap your front leg and bend your knee in a comfortable way. If today is a challenge day, you may want to lift your front heel."

**Side 1:** "The suggestion is to practice 3 breaths: As YOU breathe in, arms extend, fingers stretch wide … As YOU breathe out, release, hands on hips. (*Say 3 times* slowly.)"

**(Continue to: b./c./d.)**

**Side 2:** "From your strong warrior base, the suggestion is to move your arms in a *new* way. You can move with me as I practice shoulder rolls forward and back or move in your own *new* way. (*Cue your stretches.*) Moving to 'find your balance' builds strength." **(Continue to: b./c./d.)**

   b.  **Exalted Warrior:** "The suggestion is to add exalted warrior to your flow. With your back hand on the back hip, lift your front arm in a comfortable way. Today arcing your arm overhead may be part of your flow. Let's practice 2 more breaths here. Feel the breath in … Feel the breath out. (*Say 2 times slowly.*) When you are ready, come back to standing tall."

   c.  **'Find a New Stretch':** "Now step your feet apart and give yourself a few moments to stretch in any way that feels comfortable today. You can move with me or find your own *new* stretches. (*Cue your stretches.*) Today, you may want to gently shake it out. When you are ready, come back to standing tall."

   d.  **The 'Finger Press Breath' (see #8) (Repeat a./b./c./d. on Side 2)**

## B. Standing beside a Chair

Anything we do standing you can also do seated or even lying down.

1.  **Strengthening Flow (Side 1: a./b./c. and Side 2: a./b./c.)**

    a.  **Warrior Three (photo p. 235 (a)–(d))**

        **Warm-up:** "We always do both sides. When you are ready, put one hand on the chair. The suggestion is to slowly move your leg from side to side. A slight bend in your standing leg can protect your knee joint. If you like, move your leg in a circle, a spiral, or any comfortable way.

        1)  As YOU breathe in, lift your knee in a comfortable way. As YOU breathe out, extend that leg back until you *feel* the stretch you want today. Perhaps extend one or both arms forward.
        2)  You can put your foot down anytime; you are never stuck. If you like, hold the stretch ... but not your breath. Let's practice 2 more breaths here. Feel the breath in ... Feel the breath out. (*Say 2 times slowly.*)
        3)  When you notice your leg muscles working ... when you notice your leg muscles working, **Side 1:** wiggle your fingers. **Side 2:** press on your toes.
        4)  When you are ready, come back to standing tall." **(Continue to b./c.)**

    b.  **The 'Finger Press Breath'**

        1)  "When you are ready, gently press one shoulder back ... Then press the other shoulder back.
        2)  (*Your choice of breath fact to share.*)
        3)  If you like, put one or both hands over your heart ... Put one or both hands over your heart.
        4)  The suggestion is to practice the 'Finger Press Breath' again 3 times. As YOU breathe in, fingers press ... As YOU breathe out, release the press. (*Say 3 times slowly.*)
        5)  If you like, gently *wiggle* the fingers on one hand or shake that hand ... Then gently *wiggle* the fingers on the other hand or shake that hand. Let your hands be as still as you would like them to be."

    c.  **Tree Pose (photos p. 228, 1: (a)–(c) and 2: (a)–(c))**

**Setup:** 1) "When you are ready, turn your knee open and press your foot on the standing leg so that you feel strong today. Pressing your foot on your knee can put pressure on your knee joint.

2) Today you may want your hand on the chair. When you take it off the chair, notice again how you are 'finding your balance' and

building core strength. You can put your foot down any time; you are never stuck."

**Side 1**: "The suggestion is to practice 3 breaths. As YOU breathe in, one or both arms open wide, fingers stretch. As YOU breathe out, hands over your heart. (*Say 3 times slowly.*) When you're ready, come back to standing tall." **(Continue to: (a)/(b)/(c)/(d))**

**Side 2**: "If you like, stretch one or both arms out to the sides or overhead. The suggestion is to move in any way that makes you smile. You can move with me, or you can find your own ways to play with balance today. (*Cue your stretches.*) You can put your foot down anytime; you are never stuck." **(Continue to: (a)/(b)/(c)/(d))**

(a) **#4 Pose with a Twist**: (photos p. 232 (a), (b), (c)) "If you like, cross your ankle above the knee on your standing leg as we practice the #4 pose. Let's practice 2 breaths. Feel the breath in … Feel the breath out. (*Say 2 times slowly.*) Today you may want to create a twist. Wherever you are, let's practice 2 more breaths." (*Say 2 times slowly.*)

(b) **'Take Up Space' (Half-Moon)**: "With your hand on or off the chair, practice longer breaths in if that is comfortable, spread your fingers wide … extend your leg out to the side … as you breathe and stretch and strengthen. The suggestion is to practice 2 more longer breaths in. On YOUR next breath in, stretch out and 'Take Up Space'. As YOU breathe out, *wiggle* your fingers or toes. (*Say 2 times slowly.*) When you are ready and as *slowly* as you would like, release to standing tall."

(c) **Feel the Heartbeat**: "When you are ready, put one or both hands over your heart. When you feel your heart beating … when you feel your heart beating, switch hands."

(d) **Toe Stretches: (Stand on the other side of the chair. Repeat on Side 2: a./b./c./d.)**

2. **'Feel the Breath' – Choose Your Breathing Pattern**

   1) "When you are ready, gently press one shoulder back … Then press the other shoulder back.

   2) Long, slow breaths out *can* lower blood pressure and lower heart rate. Longer breaths in *can* be energizing.

   3) The suggestion is to practice 5 five breaths using the breathing pattern you choose today.

   Feel the breath in … Feel the breath out. (*Say 2 times slowly.*) Always breathe in a comfortable way. Feel the breath in … Feel the breath out. (*Say 3 times slowly.*)

4) If you like, gently *stretch* the fingers on one hand or shake that hand … Then gently *stretch* the fingers on the other hand or shake that hand."

3. **'Tip-to-Toe Stretch' with Leg Balance:**

## C. Seated

1. **Comfortable Seat (see above)**

2. **'The Wave Breath'** (photos p. 242 (c) and (d))

   1) "When you are ready, gently press one shoulder back … Then press the other shoulder back.
   2) (*Your choice of breath fact to share.*)
   3) The suggestion is to practice 'The Wave Breath' 5 times.

   As YOU breathe in, hands lift (*palms up*) … As YOU breathe out, release (*palms down*). (*Say 2 times slowly.*) Always breathe in a comfortable way. On YOUR next breath in, hands lift … As YOU breathe out, release. As YOU breathe in, hands lift … As YOU breathe out, release.
   (*Say last cue slowly.*)

   4) If you like, gently move the fingers on one hand or shake that hand … Then gently move the fingers on the other hand or shake that hand."

3. **Seated Shoulder Stretches (a./b./c.)** (photos p. 239 (a)–(c))

   a. **The '1-2-3' Shoulder Stretch**

      1) "When you are ready, gently bend your elbows in a comfortable way as we practice the '1-2-3' shoulder stretch.
      2) As YOU breathe in, press both shoulders back. That's 1.

      As YOU breathe out, press both shoulders forward. That's 2. And release. That's 3.

      3) The suggestion is to practice 2 more sets of the '1-2-3' shoulder stretch. (*Say slowly 2 more times.*)
      4) If you like, tap one *hand or foot* 4 times … Then tap the other *hand or foot* 4 times."

b. **Shoulder Rolls**

1) "The suggestion is to practice 3 shoulder rolls forward and 3 back.
2) As YOU breathe in, shoulders lift … As YOU breathe out, shoulders roll forward and down.

Even small stretches have benefits. (*Say 3 times slowly.*)

3) As YOU breathe in, shoulders lift … As YOU breathe out, shoulders roll back and down." (*Say 3 times slowly.*)

c. **'Find a New Stretch'**

1) "Give yourself a few moments to find a *new* way to stretch. You can move with me or perhaps find your own *new* way to move today. (*Cue your stretches.*)
2) If you like, tap your *fingertips* on your legs 4 times. Then move your *fingertips* 4 times in a new way, perhaps strumming or patting."

4. **Classic Twist with Cat/Cow** (photos p. 230 (a)–(c))

1) "We always do both sides. As you breathe in, press down on your hands. As YOU breathe out, bring your hands around to one side to create a gentle twist.
2) The suggestion is to practice 3 breaths as you find your own rhythm. As YOU breathe in, hands press. As YOU breathe out, release the press. (*Say 3 times slowly.*)
3) When you are ready, come back to facing front, hands on your legs.
4) Let's practice seated cat/cow 2 times before we twist to the other side.

Always breathe and move in a comfortable way. As YOU breathe in, chin lifts … shoulders back … rock forward. As YOU breathe out, chin tucks … shoulders forward … rock back. (*Say 2 times slowly.*)

5) When you are ready, come back to sitting tall. (**Repeat on other side.**)
6) If you like, begin to circle slowly, in any way that feels comfortable today. Give yourself time with the stretch. When you are ready, move in the other direction."

## D. 'Final Stretch' (15 minutes)

The suggestions for creating a version of 'Final Stretch' that meets your personal and professional needs are in Chapter 9 (p. 167). The downloadable clipboard script is in Appendix C.

**V. 'All Together Now' (60 minutes): This sequence supports refugee and immigrant (ESOL) groups building connections with themselves and their communities.**

This practice sequence includes the favorite simple breathwork and poses from the many classes I have taught to people from all over the world. For language considerations, ... in a way that feels *good or comfortable* today is used.

## A. Seated

**Opening Connections (10 minutes):** This time is for sharing food, introductions, and new words (see p. 179). Anything that we do standing, you can do seated. You can always find ways to breathe and move with me.

## B. Standing

1. **'Silly Shake and Stretch'**

    1) "Let's give ourselves a few minutes to do the 'Silly Shake and Stretch'. You can move gently or shake in a way that feels good or comfortable today. Find your own ways to move or follow along with me.

    2) If you like, gently *move* one hand or shake one hand ... Then gently *move* or shake the other hand. You might like to move one leg or gently shake it out. Then move or gently shake the other leg. You might *stretch* your arms toward the ceiling, or maybe today you feel like *waving* and *shaking*. If you like, *stretch* your arms out to the sides or overhead. If you like, move one shoulder and then the other. Is there something you haven't moved or shaken yet?" (*Cue your stretches for 2 minutes.*)

2. **'Feel the Breath'** (see p. 125)

    1) "When you are ready, gently press one shoulder back ... Then press the other shoulder back.
    2) (*Your choice of breath fact to share.*)
    3) The suggestion is to practice 5 breaths.
    4) Feel the breath in ... Feel the breath out. (*Say 2 times slowly.*) Always breathe in a way that feels good or comfortable. Feel the breath in ... Feel the breath out. (*Say 3 times slowly.*)
    5) If you like, gently *stretch* the fingers on one hand or shake that hand ... Then gently *stretch* the fingers on the other hand or shake that hand."

3.  **'Tip-to-Toe' Stretch**

    1) "When you are ready, stretch one arm out to the side or overhead as we do the 'Tip-to-Toe' stretch. Then stretch the other arm to the side or overhead.

    2) Find your own rhythm as you stretch one arm, fingers spread wide … Then stretch the other arm, fingers spread wide.

    3) When you are ready, come back to standing tall."

4.  **'Ring the Bell'** (photos p. 232 (a)–(c))

    1) "When you are ready, step your feet apart in any way that feels good or comfortable today. As we practice 'Ring the Bell', gently move your arms from the front to the back, tapping your low back … your mid-back … and your upper back as you move up and down your back.

    2) If you like, hold your hands in a *new* way: now either 'ring the bell' with an open palm or a closed hand. Take your time with the stretch as you gently create length in your back."

5.  **Wide-legged Add-ons** (photos p. 234 (a)–(c))

    1) "When you are ready, step your feet apart, hands on your hips.

    2) If you like, roll from the inside edges to the outside edges of your feet … Roll from the inside to the outside edges of your feet in a way that feels good or comfortable today.

    3) If you like, press one hip to one side … Then press the other hip to the other side. Find your own rhythm as you move.

    4) Perhaps gently lift and then arc one shoulder as you press your hip to one side … Then gently lift and arc the other shoulder as you press to the other side.

    5) When you are ready, come back to standing tall, hands on your hips."

    **Variation:** "Perhaps today, arc one arm and then the other overhead as you move from side to side."

6.  **Toe Stretches**

    1) "When you are ready, gently press one shoulder back … Then press the other shoulder back.

    2) If you like, with your hands still on your hips, lift one heel and press on the toes in a way that feels good or comfortable today. Then lift the other heel and press on the toes.

    3) The suggestion is to practice 2 more sets of toe stretches." (*Say 2 more times slowly.*)

## C. Seated

1. **Comfortable Seat**

   1) "Give yourself a few moments to find a way to sit that feels good or comfortable today.
   2) If you like, move from side to side as you find a comfortable seat. You may want to move in a circle. Take your time as you move.
   3) When you are ready, gently press one shoulder back … Then press the other shoulder back.
   4) If you like, tap your *hands* 4 times."

2. **'Feel the Breath'**

   1) "When you are ready, gently press one shoulder back again … Then press the other shoulder back.
   2) (*Your choice of breath fact to share.*)
   3) Put one or both hands over your heart … Put one or both hands over your heart. The suggestion is to practice 5 breaths.
   4) Feel the breath in … Feel the breath out. (*Say 2 times slowly.*) Always breathe in a way that feels good or comfortable today. Feel the breath in … Feel the breath out. (*Say 3 times slowly.*)
   5) If you like, gently *stretch* the fingers on one hand or shake that hand … Then gently *stretch* the fingers on the other hand or shake that hand."

3. **Neck and Shoulder Stretches (a./b./c./d.)**

   a. **Neck Massage (photos p. 240 (a))**

   "When you are ready, take one hand and rub the back of your neck or the fronts of your shoulders. (*Slowly cue each.*) Today you may want to:

   1) Use one or both hands.
   2) Gently tuck your chin and move your chin from side to side as you massage.
   3) Massage the base of the neck/top of the back.
   4) Gently lift and lower the chin as you massage."

   b. **Chin Lift and Release (photos p. 240 (b) and (c))**

   1) "Let's practice the chin lift and release 3 times. As YOU breathe in, chin lifts. As YOU breathe out, chin releases.
   (*Say 3 times slowly.*)
   2) With your chin still released, slowly move your chin from side to side. Take your time with the stretch."

c. **Shoulder Rolls (photos p. 238 (a) and (b))**

    1) When you are ready, the suggestion is to practice 3 shoulder rolls forward and 3 back.

    2) As YOU breathe in, shoulders lift ... As YOU breathe out, shoulders roll forward and down. (*Say 3 times slowly.*) Now 3 back.

    3) As YOU breathe in, shoulders lift ... As YOU breathe out, shoulders roll back and down." (*Say 3 times slowly.*)

d. **The '1-2-3' Stretch (photos p. 239 (a), (b), (c))**

    1) "When you are ready, gently bend your elbows in a way that feels good or comfortable today as we practice the '1-2-3' shoulder stretch.

       As YOU breathe in, press both shoulders back. That's 1. As YOU breathe out, press both shoulders forward. That's 2. And release. That's 3. Let's practice 2 more sets of the '1-2-3' shoulder stretch." (*Say slowly 2 more times.*)

4. **'Open and Close Breath'** (see p. 127)

    1) "When you are ready, gently press one shoulder back ... Then press the other shoulder back. Let's practice the 'Open and Close Breath' 5 times.

    2) As YOU breathe in, fingers move ... As YOU breathe out, release. (*Say 2 times slowly.*)

Always breathe and move in a comfortable way. On YOUR next breath in, fingers move ... As YOU breathe out, release. As YOU breathe in, fingers move ... As YOU breathe out, release. (*Repeat last cue slowly.*)

If you like, gently *move* the fingers on one hand or shake that hand ... Then gently *move* the fingers on the other hand or shake that hand."

## D. Standing

Anything we do standing, you also can do seated.

1. **Peaceful Warrior One with Counting**

    1) "We always do both sides. When you are ready, step one foot forward into our circle. Hands on hips, bend your front leg in a way that feels good or comfortable today. (The setup is a high lunge, no chair.)

2) Let's count in different languages as we practice 3 times. As YOU breathe in ... (someone says *one* in their language as arms lift). As YOU breathe out ... (Everyone says *one* in that language as arms release). (*Say 2 more times slowly.*)

3) When you are ready, come back to standing tall.

2. **'Feel the Breath'** 3 times. **(See above.) (Repeat with different language on other side.)**

3. **'Find a New Stretch'** Give yourself time to find a *new* stretch today. You may want to find some gentle stretches or to shake it out. You can follow along with me if you like." (*Cue your stretches.*)

## E. Standing (by chair)

1. **Tree Pose (Side 1: a./b. and Side 2: a./b.)** (*Strong* or *play* may be the word of the day to share in different languages.)

   a. **Tree Pose (photos p. 228, 1: (a)–(c) and 2: (a)–(c))**

   Setup: "We always do both sides. With your hand on the chair, move your leg from side to side in any way that feels good or comfortable to you today. Maybe move your leg in a circle to gently stretch the muscles.

   1) When you are ready, turn your knee open and press your foot so that you feel *strong* today.
   2) With your hand on the chair, you can focus on the stretch. When you take it off the chair, you build strength as you 'find your balance'. You can put your foot down any time; you are never stuck.

   Side 1: The suggestion is to practice 3 breaths. As YOU breathe in, one or both arms open wide, fingers stretch. On YOUR breath out, hands over your heart. (*Say 3 times slowly.*) **(Continue to b.)**

   Side 2: If you like, stretch one or both arms to the side or overhead. Move your arms in any way that makes you smile. You can move with me or find your own ways to *play* with balance today.

   3) When you are ready, come back to standing tall, hands on your hips."

   b. **Toe Stretches**

   1) "When you are ready, gently press one shoulder back ... Then press the other shoulder back.

2) If you like, lift one heel and press on the toes in a way that feels good or comfortable today. Then lift the other heel and press on the toes. The suggestion is to practice 2 more sets of toe stretches." (*Say 2 times slowly.*) **(Repeat Side 2 a./b. standing on other side of chair.)**

2. **'Kitchen Stretch' (a./b./a./c.)** (photos p. 237)

   **Setup:** "Let's practice 3 ways to protect your back anytime you bend forward: gently press shoulders back, hips back, and slightly bend knees. When you are ready, rest your hands or forearms on the back of the chair. Notice that your shoulders are back, hips are back, and knees are bent."

   a. **'Strong and Steady':** "The suggestion is to practice 4 breaths as we practice 'Strong and Steady'. As YOU breathe in, feel the press on the chair … As YOU breathe out, press hips back." (*Say 4 times slowly.*)

   b. **'Hip Rock 'n Roll':**

      1) "If you like, stand and put your hands on your hips. Give yourself a moment to practice lifting your tailbone and tucking your tailbone. Find your own rhythm as you lift and tuck in 'Hip Rock 'n Roll'.

      2) When you are ready, set up for 'Kitchen Stretch' again. (*Repeat Setup.*) On YOUR next breath in, tailbone lifts … as YOU breathe out, tailbone tucks as we practice 'Hip Rock 'n Roll'.

      3) If you like, do two more sets, finding your own rhythm as you move and breathe."

   **Repeat b. 'Strong and Steady'**

   c. **Shoulder Rolls Back:**

      1) "As you are ready, come to standing. Let's practice three shoulder rolls back.

      2) As YOU breathe in, shoulders lift … As YOU breathe out, shoulders roll back and down. (*Say 3 times slowly.*)

   Maybe next time you are in the kitchen or at work, you give yourself one minute to stretch your back."

3. **'Ring the Bell'** (see p. 221)

4. **'Tip-to-Toe' Stretch** (see p. 221)

## F. Seated

1. **Comfortable Seat** (see p. 222)
2. **'The Wave Breath'** (more on p. 129) (see p. 242 (c) and (d))

   1) "When you are ready, gently press one shoulder back … Then press the other shoulder back.
   2) (*Your choice of breath fact to share.*)
   3) The suggestion is to practice 'The Wave Breath' 5 times.

      As YOU breathe in, hands lift (*palms up*) … As YOU breathe out, release (*palms down*). (*Say 2 times slowly.*) Always breathe in a comfortable way. On YOUR next breath in, hands lift … As YOU breathe out, release. As YOU breathe in, hands lift … As YOU breathe out, release. (*Repeat last cue slowly.*)

   4) If you like, gently *stretch* the fingers on one hand or shake that hand … Then gently *stretch* the fingers on the other hand or shake that hand.
   5) What could we call this breath?"

3. **Favorites**

"What stretch or breath would you like to do again?" You can either ask for volunteers, depending on time – let's have 3 ideas (always set a time boundary) – or go around the circle. If someone does not want to share today, let them know to simply look to the next person. Sometimes people are not comfortable volunteering (drawing attention to themselves), but they will share an idea if it is their turn.

4. **Twist with Cat-Cow** (photos p. 230 (a)–(c))

   1) "When you are ready, gently press one shoulder back … Then press the other shoulder back. If you like, tap your *fingertips* on your legs.
   2) We always do both sides. On YOUR next breath in, press down on your hands. As YOU breathe out, bring your hands around to one side.
   3) The suggestion is to practice 4 breaths as you find your own rhythm. As YOU breathe in, hands press. As YOU breathe out, release the press. (*Say 4 times slowly.*)
   4) When you are ready, come back to facing front. If you like, tap your *hands* on your legs.
   5) Before we do the other side, let's practice seated cat-cow 2 times. Always move and breathe in a way that feels good or comfortable today.

As YOU breathe in, chin lifts … shoulders back … rock forward.
As YOU breathe out, chin tucks … shoulders forward … rock back.
(*Say 2 times slowly.*)

6)   When you are ready, come back to sitting tall." **(Repeat 1–6 on the other side.)**


## G. 'Make a Plan'

Give yourself a few moments to make a two-minute plan to use later when you want to change how you are feeling. The suggestion is to choose one breath we did today: we did (list breaths). A long, slow breath out *can* lower blood pressure.

If you like, add one stretch – perhaps the 'Kitchen Stretch' or the 'Tip-to-Toe' stretch. You now have a two-minute plan to do at home or at work when you want to change how you are feeling.

**********

**To Recap:** This chapter provides the trauma-informed resources needed to teach a variety of yoga breaks and practices in a variety of settings. Easy-to-use charts of phrases to empower, to build body awareness, and to build breath awareness can strengthen your trauma-informed program. Clear descriptions and suggested applications (clinical and teaching) for all the breaks and practice sequences are listed. Scripts for the practice sequences are provided. Groups of photographs (options and adaptations) support your developing a program to meet someone where they are. Finally, many resource materials are downloadable to support your teaching efforts.

## Practice Sequence Photographs

### Tree Pose

Side 1                    Side 2

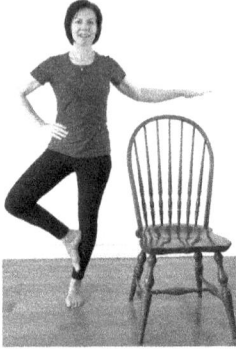
(a)

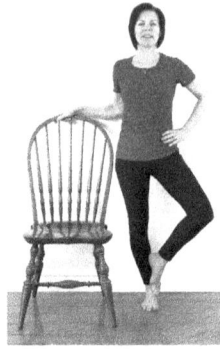
(a)

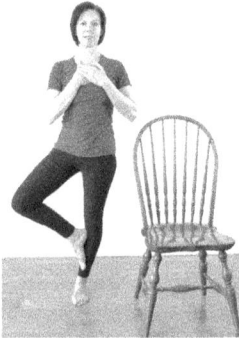
(b)

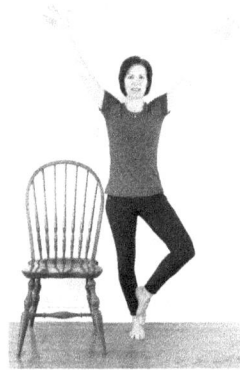
(b)

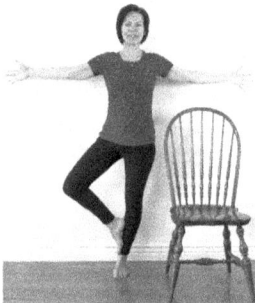
(c)

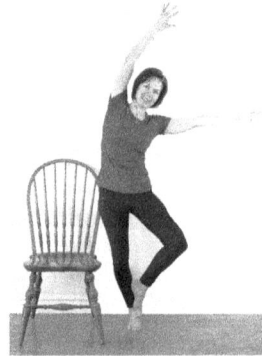
(c)

Eagle

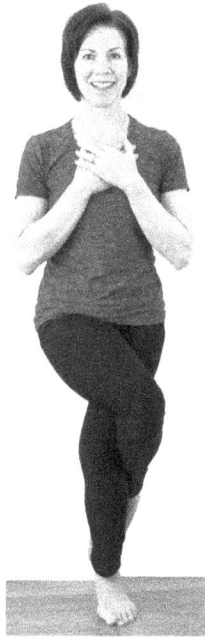

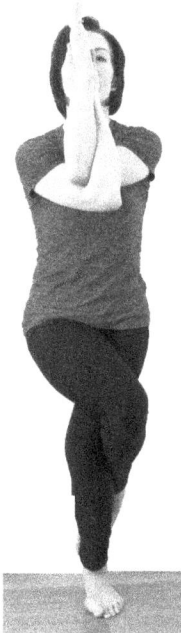

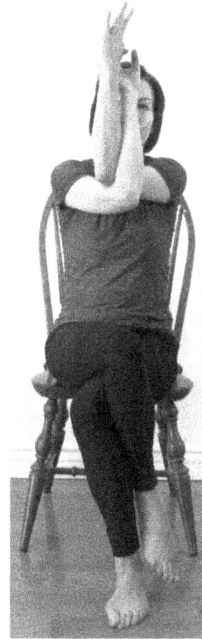

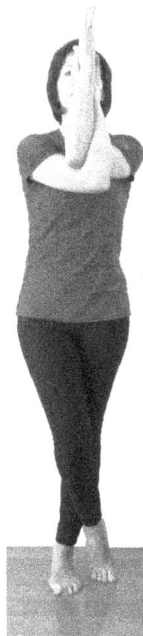

## 'Take up Space'

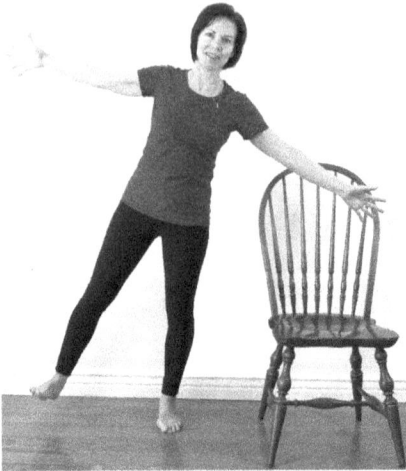

(a)

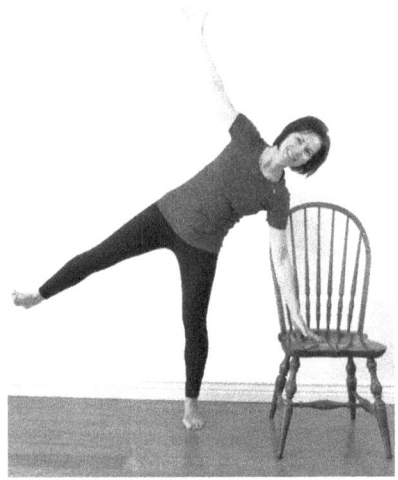

(b)

## Seated Twist with Cat/Cow

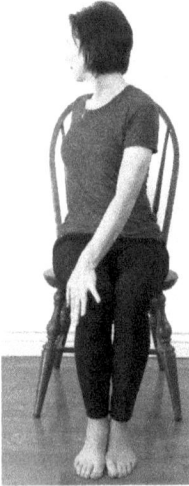

(a)

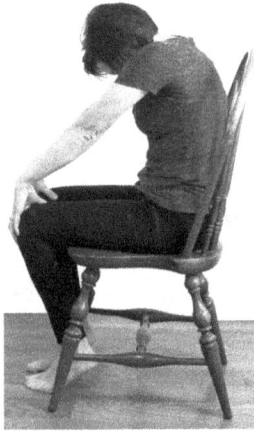

(b)

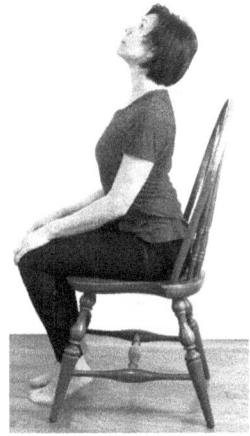

(c)

# Tip-to-Toe

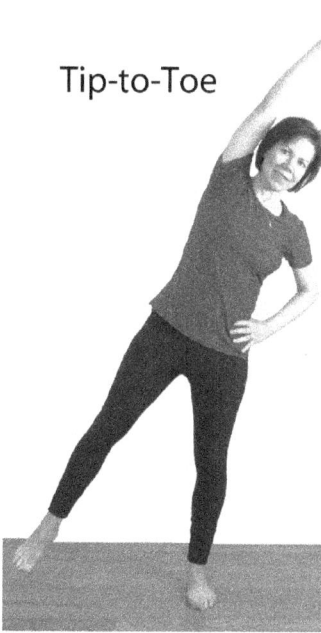

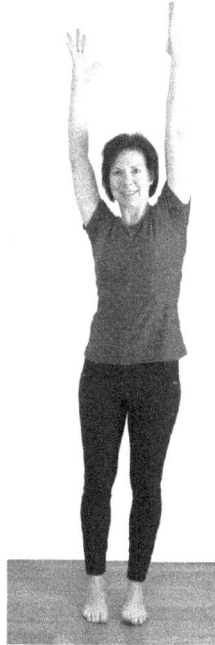

(a)

(b)

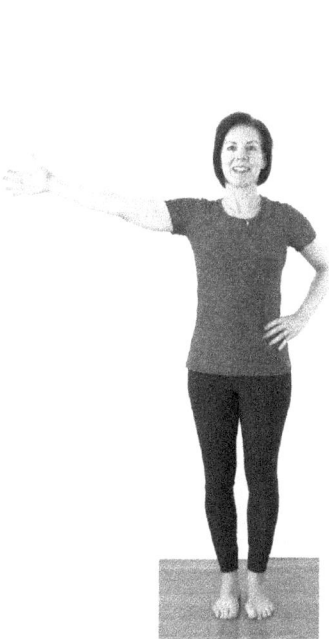

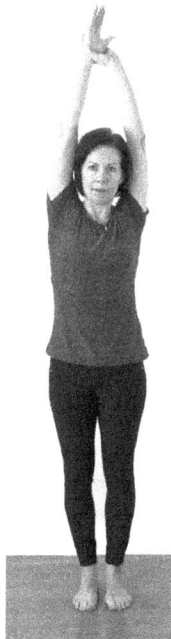

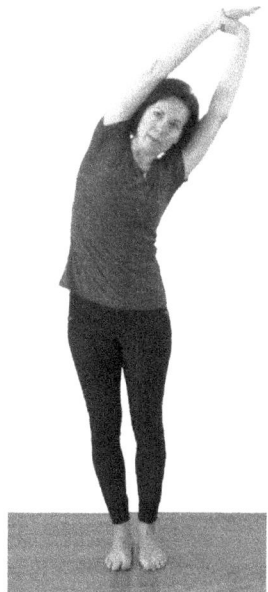

(c)

(d)

(e)

## #4 Stretch

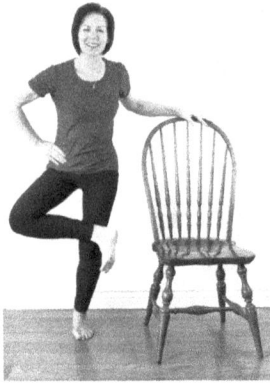 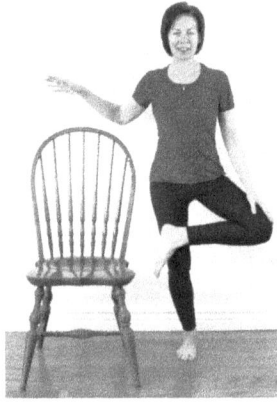 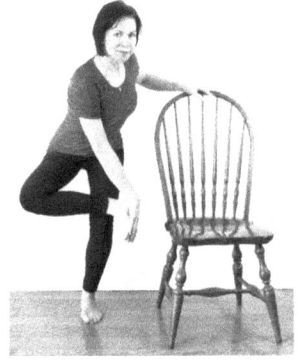

(a)                                    (b)                                    (c)

## 'Ring the Bell'

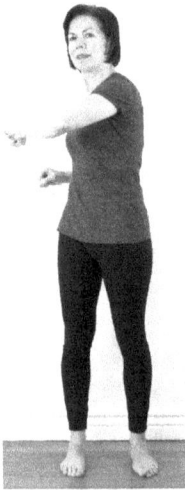 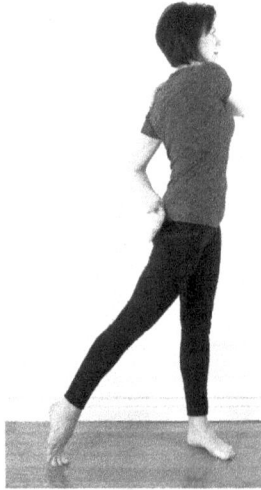 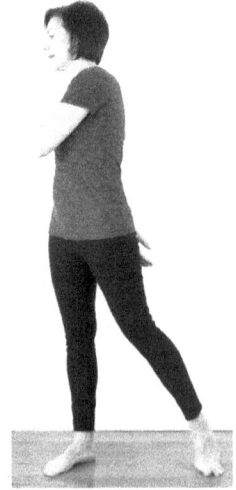

(a)                                    (b)                                    (c)

## Warrior 2 Flow

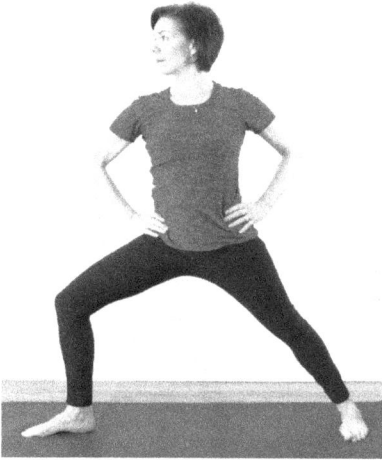

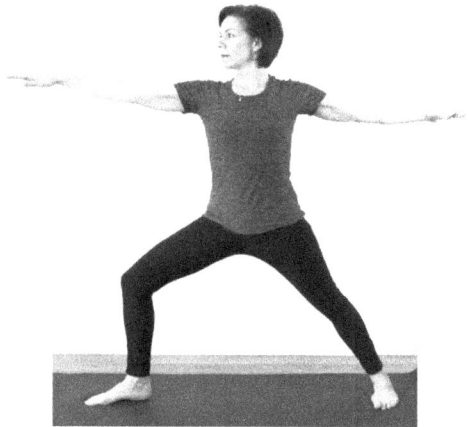

## Exalted Warrior

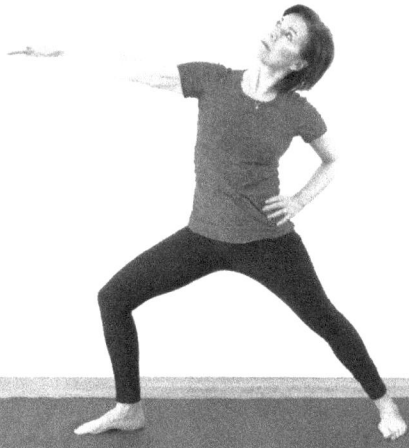

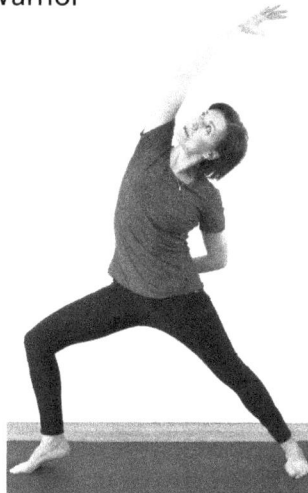

## Wide-legged Add-on

Edges of Feet

Crescent

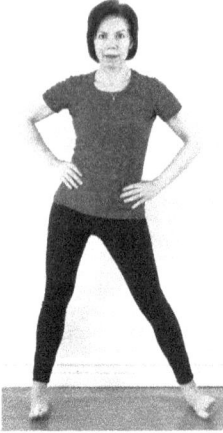

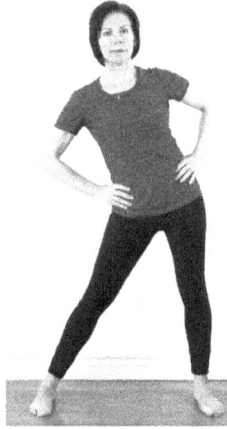

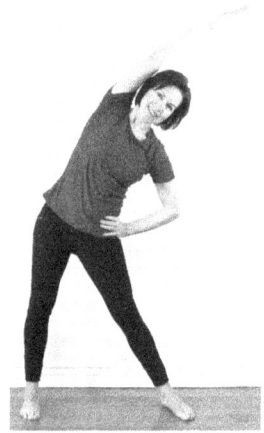

Hips to Side
(b)

(a)

(c)

## Hip & Core Strengthening 1

### Pendulum

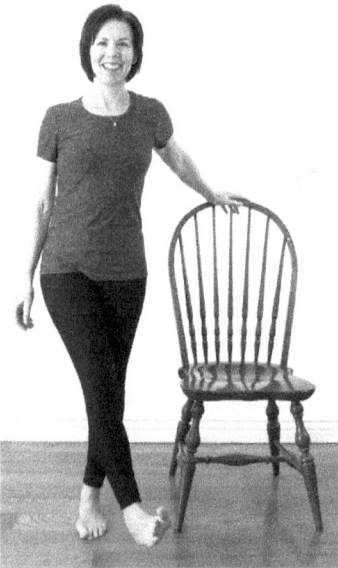

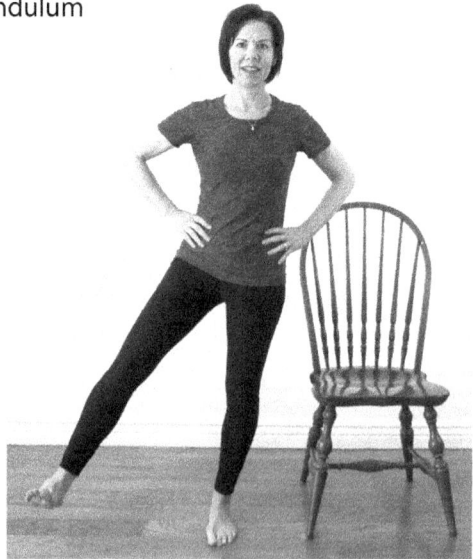

(a)

(b)

# Hip & Core Strengthening 2

Warrior 3 Flow

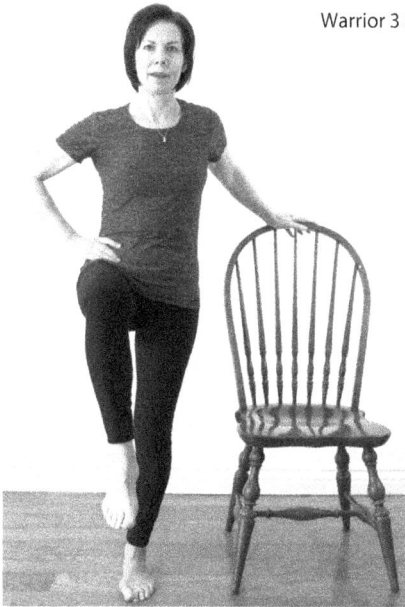

(a)

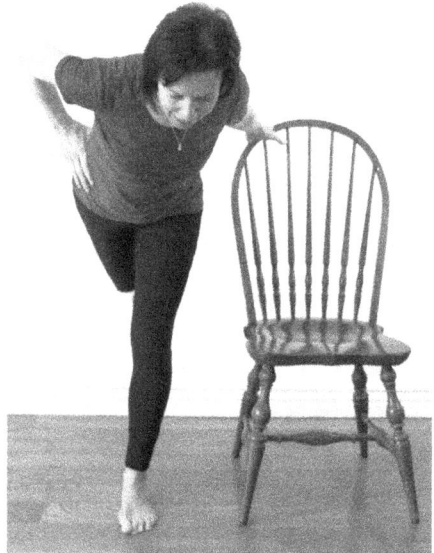

(b)

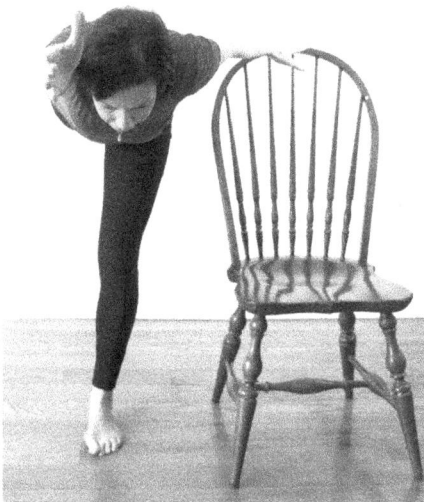

(c)

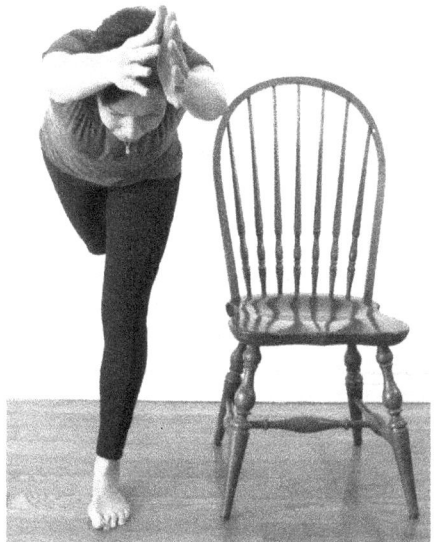

(d)

## Chair Pose Flow

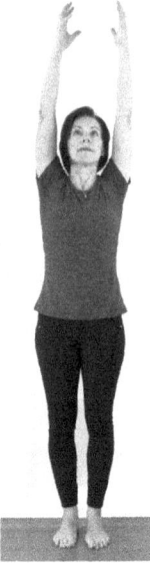

(a)

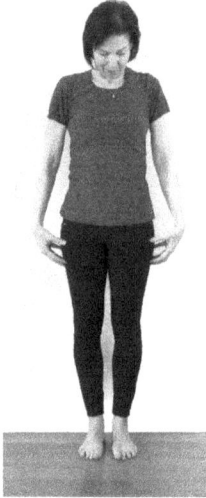

(b)

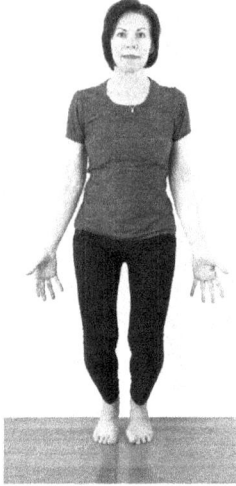

(c)

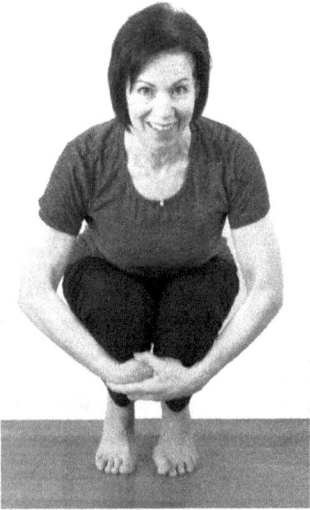

(d)

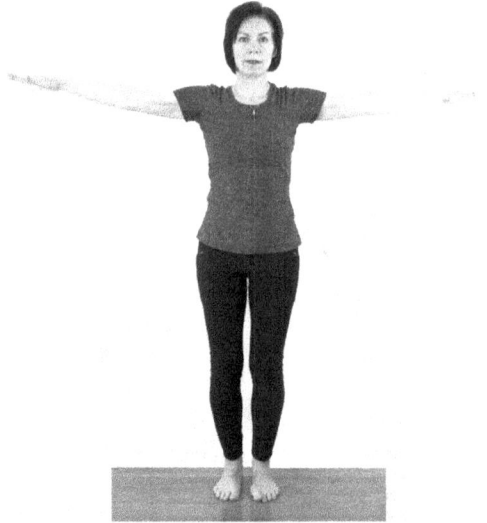

(e)

# 'Kitchen Stretch' 1

## Setup

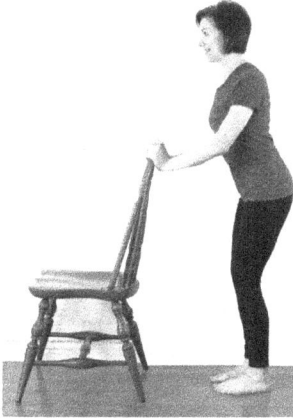
(a)

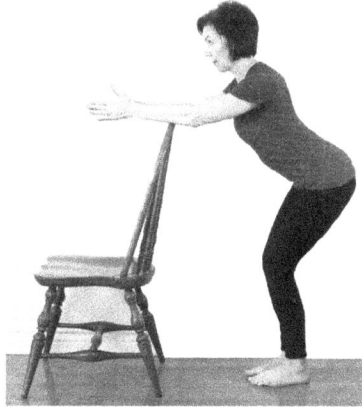
(b)

### 'Strong & Steady'

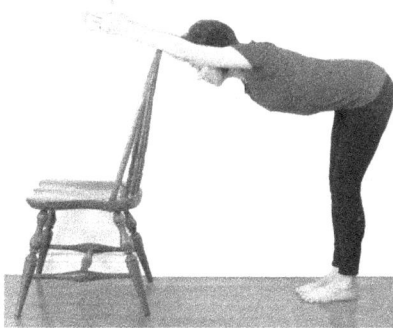
(c)

### 'Hip Rock 'n Roll'

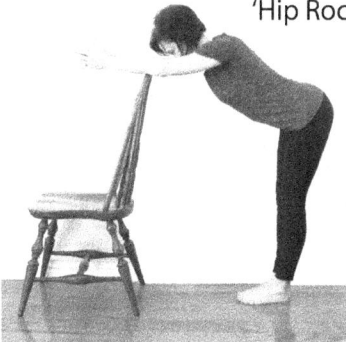
(d)

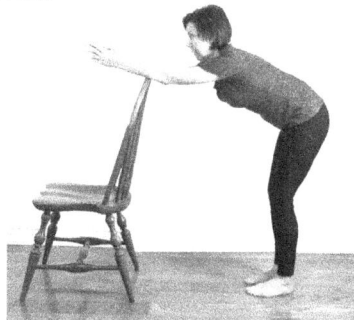
(e)

# Kitchen Stretch 2

## Psoas & Glute Stretches

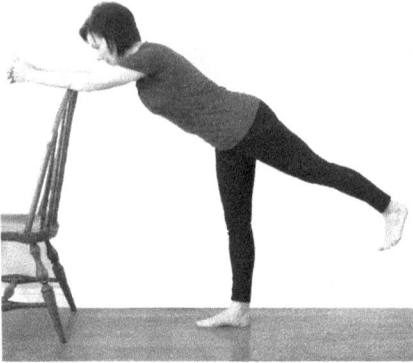
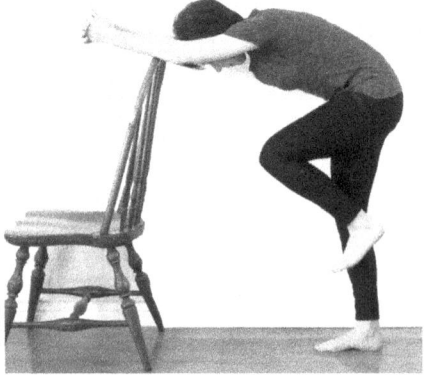

(a)                                           (b)

## Shoulder Rolls

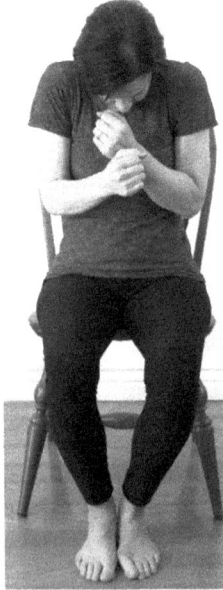
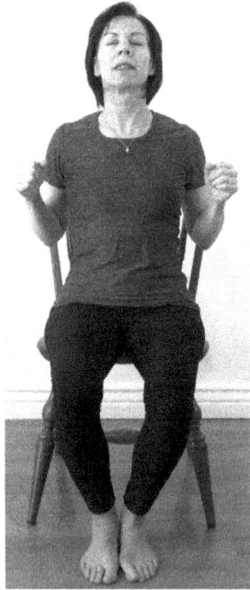

(a)                                           (b)

# Shoulder Stretches
## '1-2-3' Stretch

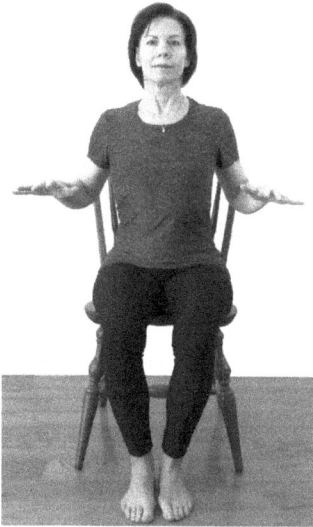
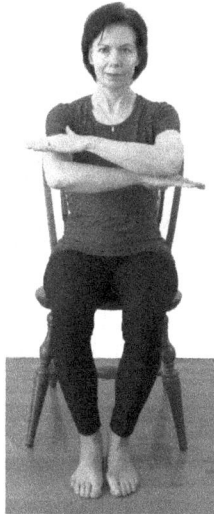
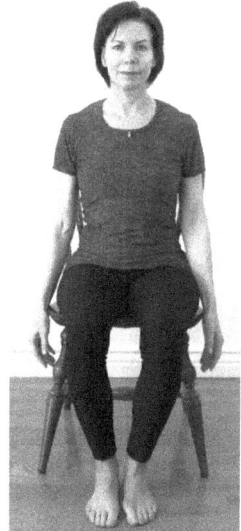

(a)                    (b)                    (c)

'Shoulder
Rock 'n Roll'

Find Own
Stretch

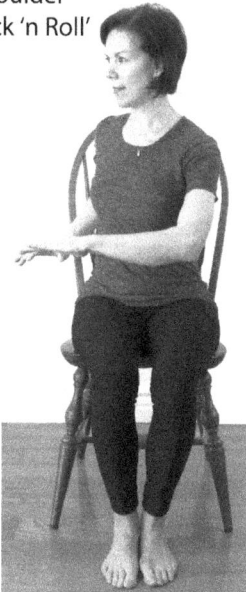
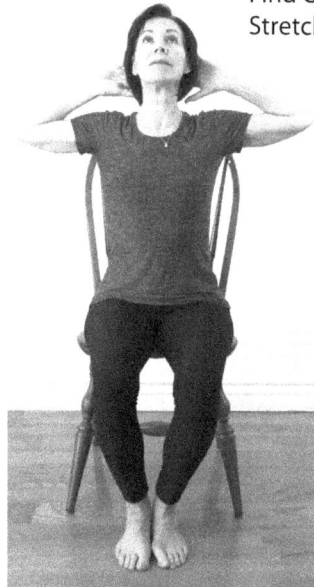

(d)                    (e)

# 'Neck & Shoulder Suite'

Neck Massage

Chin Lift
& Release

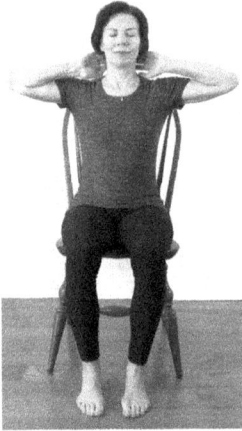

(a)

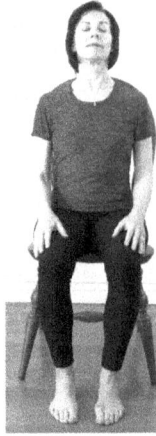

(b)

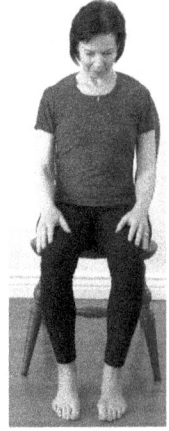

(c)

Pendulum

Head Tilt

Shoulder Roll

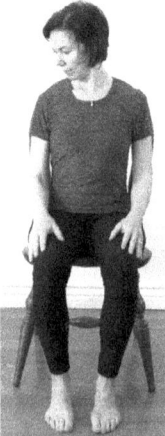

(d)

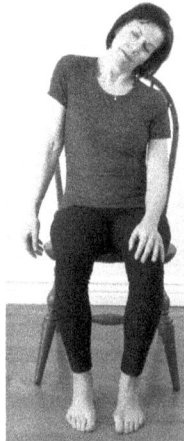

(e)

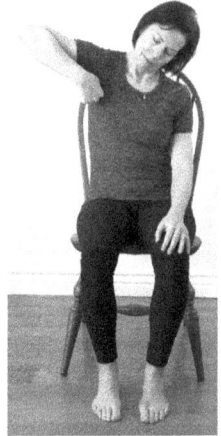

(f)

# Breathwork

### 'Goal Post Breathing'

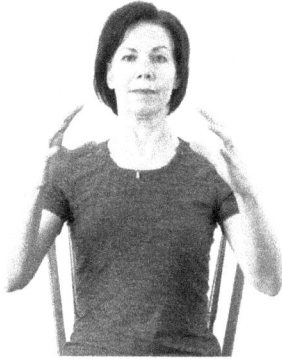

(a)

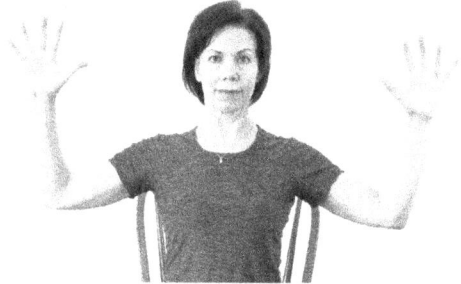

(b)

'It's a Wrap'

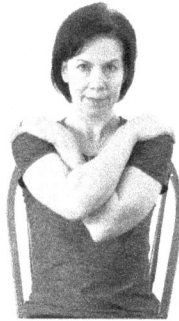

(c)

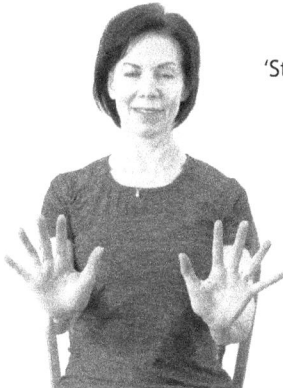

'Stop Sign Breath'

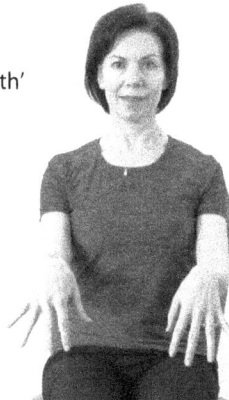

(a)                                    (b)

Many thanks to Elizabeth Q. Finlinson, LCSW
for being our yoga model.

# Breathwork

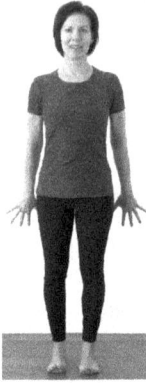

Shifting
Breath

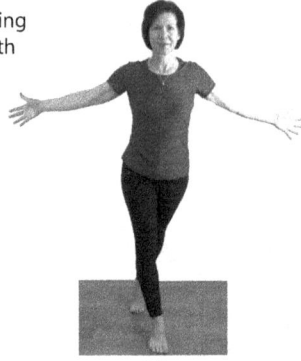

(a)                              (b)

'The Wave Breath'

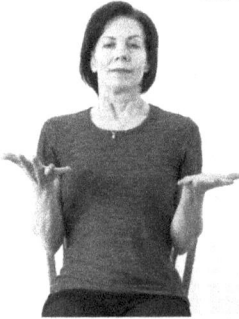

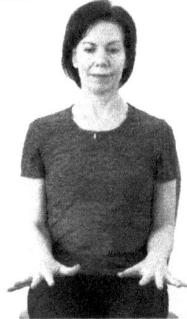

(c)                              (d)

'Anytime,
Anywhere Breath'

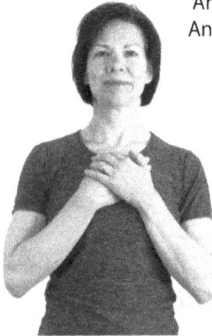

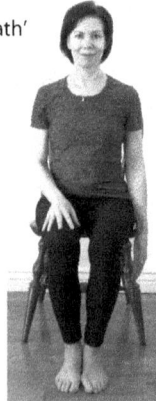

'Feel the Breath'

(e)                              (f)

# Appendix A

## Practice Scripts for Chapter 5

1) 'Tip to Toe' Stretch; 2) Wide-legged Add-on; 3) Tree Pose and Toe Stretches; 4) 'Feel the Breath'; 5) Shoulder Rolls; 6) 'Stop Sign Breath'; 7) 'Anytime, Anywhere Breath'

1. **'Tip-to-Toe' Stretch** (photos p. 231 (a)–(e))

   1) "Anything that we do standing, you can do seated. When you are ready, stretch one arm to the side or overhead as we do the 'Tip-to-Toe' stretch. Then stretch the other arm to the side or overhead.
   2) Find your own rhythm as you stretch one arm, fingers spread wide … Then stretch the other arm, fingers spread wide.
   3) If you like, grasp one wrist as you gently stretch forward or over your head. When you are ready, grasp the other wrist as you gently stretch the other arm.
   4) When you are ready, come back to standing tall, hands on your hips."

2. **Wide-legged Add-on** (photos p. 234 (a)–(c))

   1) "When you are ready, step your feet apart in a comfortable way. Put your hands on your hips.
   2) If you like, roll from the inside edges to the outside edges of your feet … Roll from the inside to the outside edges of your feet.
   3) In whatever way feels comfortable today, press one hip to one side … Then press the other hip to the other side. Find your own rhythm as you move.
   4) You may like to gently lift and then arc one shoulder as you press your hip to one side … Then gently lift and arc the other shoulder as you press to the other side.
   5) When you are ready, come back to standing tall."

3. **Tree Pose (standing by chair)** (photos p. 228 (a)–(f))

**Setup:**

1) "We always do both sides. When you are ready, turn your knee open and press your foot against your standing leg so that you feel *strong* today. Pressing your foot on the knee can put pressure on your knee joint.
2) Today you may want your hand on the chair. When you take it off the chair, notice how you are 'finding your balance' and building core strength. You can put your foot down any time; you are never stuck.

**Side 1:** The suggestion is to practice 3 breaths. As YOU breathe in, one or both arms open wide, fingers stretch. As YOU breathe out, hands over your heart." (*Say 3 times slowly.*)

(Stand other side of chair for side 2.)

**Side 2:** "If you like, lift one or both arms to the side or overhead. Move your arms in any way that makes you smile. You can move with me or find your own ways to *play* with balance. Today you may move your arms in a *new* way, simply noticing how they are moving."

(Practice Toe stretches.)

**Toe Stretches**

1) "The suggestion is to come back to standing tall, hands on your hips.
2) When you are ready, gently press one shoulder back … Then press the other shoulder back.
3) If you like, lift one heel and press on the toes in a way that feels comfortable today. Then lift the other heel and press on the toes. The suggestion is to practice 2 more sets of toe stretches."
(*Say 2 times slowly.*)

4. **'Feel the Breath'**

1) "When you are ready, gently press one shoulder back … Then press the other shoulder back.
2) Long, slow breaths out *can* lower heart rate and lower blood pressure.
3) If you like, put one or both hands over your heart … Put one or both hands over your heart.

The suggestion is to practice 5 five breaths.

4) Feel the breath in … Feel the breath out. (*Say 2 times slowly.*) Always breathe in a comfortable way. Feel the breath in … Feel the breath out. (*Say 3 times slowly.*)

5) If you like, gently *stretch* the fingers on one hand or shake that hand … Then gently *stretch* the fingers on the other hand or shake that hand. Let your hands be as still as you would like them to be."

## 5. Shoulder Rolls

1) "The suggestion is to practice 3 shoulder rolls forward and 3 back.

2) As YOU breathe in, shoulders lift … As YOU breathe out, shoulders roll forward and down. (*Say 3 times slowly.*)

3) As YOU breathe in, shoulders lift … As YOU breathe out, shoulders roll back and down. (*Say 3 times slowly.*)

4) When you are ready, move your shoulders so you feel a *new* stretch. You can move with me or move in any way that feels comfortable to you today. (*Slowly cue what you are doing.*)

5) If you like, tap your *hands* on your legs 4 times."

## 6. 'Stop Sign Breath' (photos p. 241 (d) and (e))

1) "When you are ready, gently press one shoulder back … Then press the other shoulder back.

2) (*No breath fact.*)

3) The suggestion is to practice the 'Stop Sign Breath' 5 times.

As YOU breathe in, palms press forward, (ONLY *you softly say 'stop'*) … As YOU breathe out, fingers down. (*Say 2 times slowly.*) Always move and breathe in a comfortable way.

On YOUR next breath in, palms press forward, (*stop*) … As YOU breathe out, fingers down.

As YOU breathe in, palms forward, (*stop*) … As YOU breathe out, fingers down. (*Repeat last cue slowly.*)

4) If you like, gently *wiggle* the finger on one hand or shake that hand, then gently *wiggle* the fingers on the other hand or shake that hand."

## 7. 'Anytime, Anywhere Breath' (photos p. 242 (f))

1) You can do the 'Anytime, Anywhere Breath' seated or standing, eyes open eyes closed, in a group, and even when you are talking with someone.

2) "When you are ready, gently press one shoulder back … Then press the other shoulder back. If you like, place one hand on your leg.

3) The suggestion is to take long, slow breaths out if that is comfortable today.

4) Let's practice 5 breaths. As YOU breathe in, fingers press … As YOU breathe out, release. (*Say 2 times slowly.*) Always breathe in a comfortable way. On YOUR next breath in, fingers press … As YOU breathe out, release. As YOU breathe in, fingers press … As YOU breathe out, release. (*Repeat last cue slowly.*)

5) When you are ready, gently *move* the fingers on one hand or shake that hand … Then gently *move* the fingers on the other hand or shake that hand."

# Appendix B
## Resources

These resources have shaped the GreenTREE Yoga® Approach.

## Books and Audio Books

### Breathing

Kahn, S. and Erlich, P. (2018). *Jaws: The Story of A Hidden Epidemic.* Stanford University Press.

Nestor, J. (2020). *Breath: The New Science of a Lost Art.* Riverhead Books.

### Compassion Fatigue/Vicarious Trauma

Mathieu, F. (2011). *The Compassion Fatigue Workbook: Creative Tools for Transforming Compassion Fatigue and Vicarious Traumatization.* Routledge Press.

Van Dernoot Lipsky, L. and Burk, C. (2009). *Trauma Stewardship: An Everyday Guide to Caring for Self While Caring for Others.* Berrett-Koehler Publishers.

### Mindfulness

Bell, C. (2016). *Mindful Yoga, Mindful Life: A Guide for Everyday Practice.* Shambhala Press.

Kornfield, J. (2008). *The Wise Heart.* Bantam Books.

### Movement

Feldenkrais, M. (reprint 2019). *Awareness Through Movement: Easy-to-Do Health Exercises to Improve Your Posture, Vision, Imagination, and Personal Awareness.* HarperOne.

Feldenkrais, M. (1981/2019). *The Elusive Obvious: The Convergence of Movement, Neuroplasticity and Health*. North Atlantic Press.

Ratey, J. (2018/2013). *Spark: The Revolutionary New Science of Exercise and the Brain*. Little, Brown.

## Neuroscience/Neuroplasticity

Doidge, N. (2016). *The Brain's Way of Healing: Remarkable Discoveries and Recoveries from the Frontiers of Neuroplasticity*. Penguin Books.

Doidge, N. (2007). *The Brain That Changes Itself*. Viking Books.

Eagleman, D. (2020). *Livewired: The Inside Story of the Ever-Changing Brain*. Pantheon.

Lembke, A. (2021). *Dopamine Nation: Finding Balance in the Age of Indulgence*. Dutton.

Lieberman, D. Z. and Long, M. D. (2019). *The Molecule of More: How a Single Chemical in Your Brain Drives Love, Sex, and Creativity–And Will Determine the Fate of the Human Race*. BenBella Books.

Merzenich, M. (2013). *Soft-wired: How the New Science of Brain Plasticity Can Change Your Life*. Parnassus Publishing.

Porges, S. (2017). *The Pocket Guide to the Polyvagal Theory: The Transformative Power of Feeling Safe*. W.W. Norton.

Porges, S. (2021). *Polyvagal Safety: Attachment, Communication, Self-Regulation (IPNB)* W.W. Norton.

Sapolsky, R. (2018). *Behave: The Biology of Humans at Our Best and Worst*. Penguin Books.

Siegel, D. (2020). *The Developing Mind: How Relationships and the Brain Interact to Shape Who We Are*, 3rd edition. The Guilford Press.

## Trauma

Calhoun, Y. (2024). *Trauma-informed Yoga for Pain Management: A Practical Manual for Simple Stretching, Gentle Strengthening, and Mindful Breathing*. Singing Dragon.

Levine, P. (2015). *Trauma and Memory: Brain and Body in a Search for the Living Past*. North Atlantic Books.

Murthy, V. H. (2020). *Together: The Healing Power of Human Connection in a Sometimes Lonely World*. Harper Wave.

Ogden, P. (2006). *Trauma and the Body: A Sensorimotor Approach to Psychotherapy*. W.W. Norton.

The Prison Yoga Project (books for incarcerated people). *Yoga a Path for Healing and Recovery, and Freedom from the Inside, a Woman's Yoga Practice Guide.* (www.prisonyoga.org)

Van der Kolk, B. (2015). *The Body Keeps the Score: Brain, Mind, and Body in the Healing of Trauma.* Penguin Publishing.

## Podcasts

Huberman Lab podcasts (https://hubermanlab.com/category/podcast-episodes/)

1) How to Breathe Correctly for Optimal Health, Mood, Learning and Performance
2) Master Stress: Tools for Managing Stress and Anxiety
3) Control Pain and Health Faster with Your Brain
4) Master Your Breathing with Dr. Jack Feldman

## Programs with resources/podcasts/links/studies

Adverse Childhood Experiences (ACEs): Information on trauma across the lifespan. https://www.cdc.gov/violenceprevention/aces/index.html

Trauma Research Foundation. Bessel van der Kolk, M.D. https://traumaresearchfoundation.org/

Sensorimotor Psychotherapy Institute®, Pat Ogden, PhD. https://sensorimotorpsychotherapy.org/

Somatic Experiencing® Peter Levine, PhD. https://www.somaticexperiencing.com/

Tend Academy: Education and Resources for Helping Professionals. https://www.tendacademy.ca/

Laura van Dernoot Lipsky: https://traumastewardship.com/laura-van-dernoot-lipsky/

# Appendix C

## Supplemental Resources
www.greentreeyoga.org/buildingsafety

---

1. Clipboard Sheets for Five Practice Sequences
2. Practice Scripts for Chapter 5
3. The 'Brain Bonus' (Transcripts, MP3s, MP4s)
4. Handouts
   a. Post-class Evaluation Form
   b. How to Find a Trauma-informed Yoga Class
   c. Benefits of Yoga
   d. Tree Pose at Home to Build Balance
5. GreenTREE Yoga®: Short Yoga Breaks: Scripts/Handouts/MP3s/MP4s
6. Sample Class Flyers
7. The PROQOL 5 Survey (Self-care)

# Index

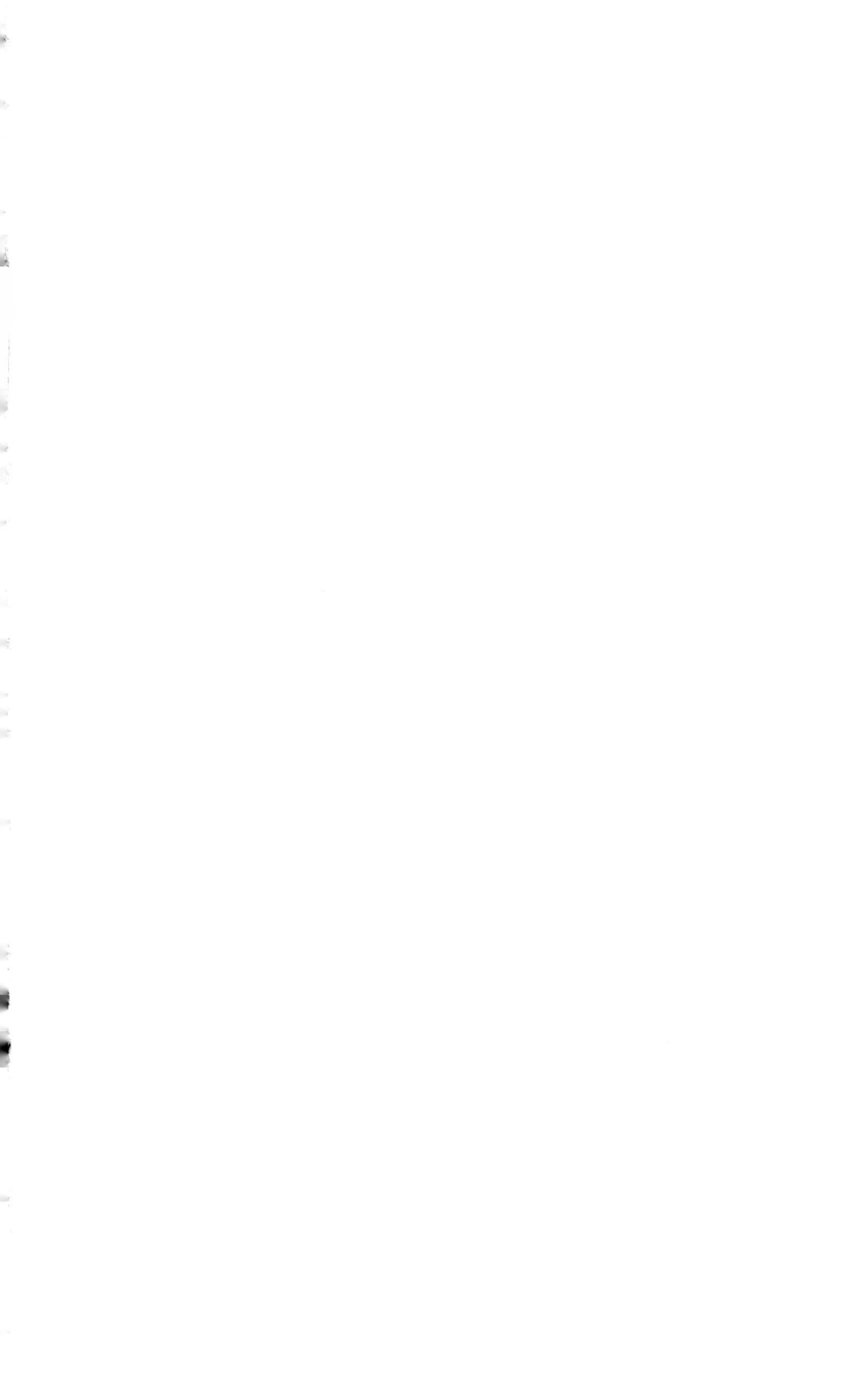

For Product Safety Concerns and Information please contact our EU
representative GPSR@taylorandfrancis.com
Taylor & Francis Verlag GmbH, Kaufingerstraße 24, 80331 München, Germany

www.ingramcontent.com/pod-product-compliance
Lightning Source LLC
Chambersburg PA
CBHW050635280326
41932CB00015B/2647